Creating a Green Home
Planning and Design

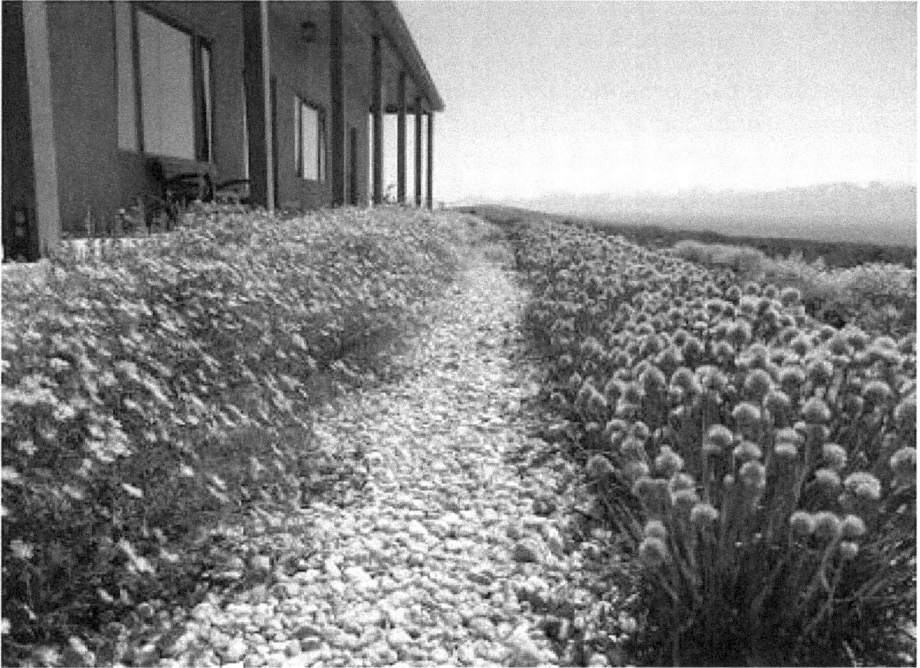

Shannon Scott
With Robert Pogoda

Catalogued in the Library of Congress 2011, originally titled: The Owner-Builder Handbook: Designing and Building with Zero Hired Help

"The soil is the great connector of lives, the source and destination of all. It is the healer and restorer and resurrector, by which disease passes into health, age into youth, death into life. Without proper care for it we can have no community, because without proper care for it we can have no life."

from *The Art of the Common Place*, *Wendell Berry*

*For those who know they can.
And for those who wonder "What if…?" and have
the will to make ifs happen.*

Table of Contents

Introduction

Creating a Green Home intends to be a reliable home building reference series for designing and constructing energy efficient, environmentally sound, healthy, and beautiful homes - with or without hired help. This book is written for those with and without any prior construction experience.

The first in the three part *Creating a Green Home* series, *Planning and Design* helps anyone thinking about building or remodeling a green home to get started. It explains and walks readers through planning steps and the why of design.

Creating a Green Home is written for owner-builders by owner builders, who have a desire to keep things simple and straight forward. We've made every effort to be thorough, yet brief and clear, so you can design and ultimately build.

For those with the means or desire to architects and contractors, this volume will give you an eye to sound energy-wise, green design concepts, and help make you a more effective site manager in that you will be able to oversee subcontractors and have a clue as to what they are doing – or should be doing. From a project's onset, most of us are filled with optimism and energy. Building a home is exciting.

However, during any building process there are headaches, dilemmas, and hardships encountered along the way. Parts or materials don't arrive when you need them. There's the constant struggle to keep straw bales covered from wet weather conditions. Winter weather often makes working outside miserable and painful. Summer heat drains us of energy and creates irritability.

The bottom line in building a home, especially for those who live rurally with few neighbors, is that building by oneself with straw or anything else is hard work and slow going. However, the rewards are numerous and lasting. Headaches fade. Storms calm. With grit and perseverance, the home gets built. Depending upon a home's size and complexity you might be facing a multi-year project. The actual design of the home primarily featured in this book took more than two years; construction from excavation to moving in, took three years. I worked full time as a teacher, but every night, weekend, holiday, and days off were spent building – even during single digit Fahrenheit winter nights. My husband, Rob, a carpenter and home inspector, worked on our home's construction full time. We hired no one.

Plan realistically. With rare exception home builders encounter delays due to weather, materials not arriving on time, and logistical problems.

If, or when, you shop for hired help, don't always go with the lowest bidder or the person who states that they'll have the work completed in record time. The delays I mentioned apply to everyone. Build quality, take your time, and don't be in a huge hurry.

Lastly, I want to alleviate any reluctance or trepidation about taking on a project of this magnitude. I want to help you do something great – design and build your own home with your own two hands. Nothing worthwhile is done easily, and the greatest satisfaction often comes from the greatest personal investments. Fear not, and venture forth. You will be fine, and your home will be fabulous.

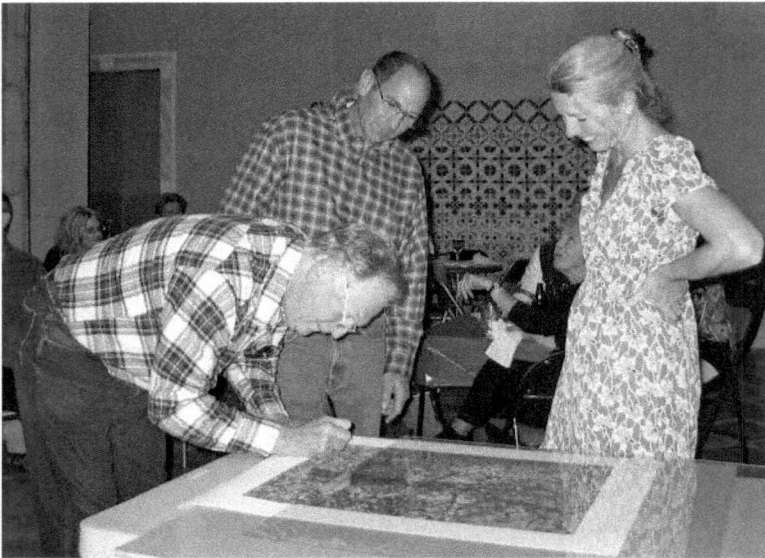

October 2008, in our nearly competed home: Rob and I (standing) as our friend Ken signs our wedding ketubah or marriage contract. We felt that if we could build a house together we could likely make a marriage work - so far so good.

Note: This planning and design volume is concise in that assumes readers have some background as to what is environmentally responsible, healthful, and what makes sound economic sense.

Part I

Planning and Design

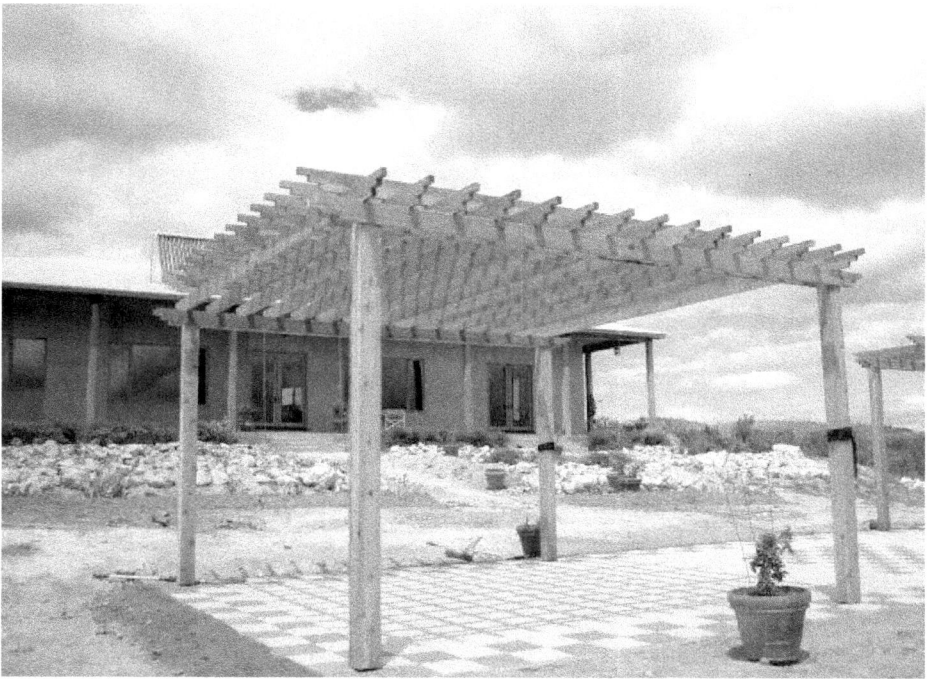

Shadows from pergolas mimic the concrete paver pattern for a geometric mirror effect incorporating art into a functional structural design.

Chapter 1

Site Selection

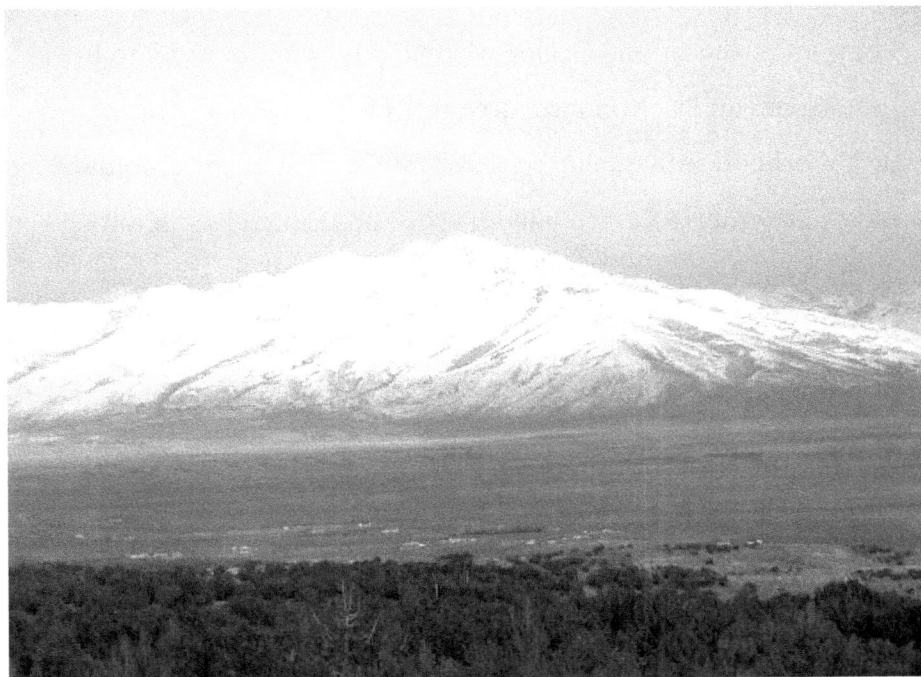

Just one of the views from our rural western building site

The first step in designing and building a house is to find a place to build it. A home must be designed to suit its site. Where you decide to build and how the home is oriented on the land will have dramatic effects upon mental and physical comfort, as well as your pocket book. You'll want to be 100% satisfied with the setting as it will tie structure to site, impact energy efficiency, and connect those who inhabit it to a place called home. Place matters.

Make a list of what you want to do in and around your home and its location. Decide whether you want, or need, to live in town or rurally. Minimize driving. Do you need an area or neighborhood with quality schools? Make a list of the absolute must have criteria for you building site and then go land scouting – which can be an enjoyable set of outings. You may see places that make you alter your list of criteria. Once you find the perfect place, remember the first rule of real estate purchase: never fall in love. You want your land for a deal, so if the price isn't right keep looking, there are always more parcels out there that will meet your needs.

Micro-Climates and Topography

Siting a home to garner as much southern exposure as possible is the single most energy-wise action an owner-builder may make in creating a home that's comfortable and pleasing to inhabit. It's also the single largest energy-wise option for most situations. If you live in the U.S. or northern hemisphere select a building site openly exposed to the south. If you are south of the equator, shop for north facing building spaces. If directionally challenged buy a good compass or global positioning system (GPS) to orient yourself with the cardinal directions.

True south and magnetic south differ by about 15°. A compass reads magnetic south, a GPS will read true. If the compass is reading 180° south, then true south will be about 195°, but check local latitude or internet source to be certain for a specific geographic location.

It's a good idea to obtain a solid feel for the potential building site by spending time on it. Camp or visit often. Look where shadows fall at noon. Determine prevailing wind and storm directions. If it's a larger parcel of land walk the terrain over and over to decide where a home would feel and function best. If the parcel affords views, garner them. If the land rests in a congested or urban area perhaps privacy is paramount so determine how a home should be placed, where bedroom windows should be, and so forth.

Do not buy or build where tall buildings or neighborhood trees may block sun from hitting the house, now or in the future. A home that receives too little sun will be colder, less cheery, use more artificial light and energy, and have limited solar applications. The home just won't feel good nor will it be energy efficient or economically sound.

Similarly, if a potential building site is nestled low near or drainage system, where cold winter air settles, the home will require more energy to keep warm during winter months. Generally, don't buy land and build next to a river, stream, lake or other low drainage, or where human activities, such as larger developments, may negatively affect riparian areas, and don't build on top of a mountain or peak of a hill where the home will be prone to winds and storms from all directions with little protection.

Select a site with sustainability and longevity in mind. That is, land that is stable in terms of geophysical features and a place you will stay for many years. Avoid land or parcels that are within a 100 year flood plain, directly on seismic faults, or where water and soil quality may be tainted. What industries are in the immediate area? Is the outdoor air and soil quality generally good? Will this site provide what you need for many years in terms of access to work, schools for children, entertainment, and outdoor recreation?

Consider the terrain's micro-climatic possibilities. For example a home that is close to an ocean shoreline will be greatly affected by offshore breezes and coastal fogs. A parcel of land farther away from the shore on a hillside may be spared colder coastal fog.

We discovered that our lot, on a rise several miles away west of a mountain range, is significantly warmer in winter and receives slightly less precipitation than parcels lower and closer to the mountains. Cold air swoops off cold mountain ridges, drops into drainage areas, then as the air warms and rises it reaches us. Consequently, we have a about a full growing season more than land in the lower drainage elevations or abutted next to the mountains.

If you like peace, quiet, and solitude, is the potential building site in a neighborhood full of teens or small children? Is it off of a main thoroughfare to commercial entities? Do you have small children and want playmates for them? If you detest driving to work or to buy groceries, look for a lot in a community area with services within cycling or walking distance. If you are nearing retirement or are retired, work from home, or other life situations where driving is less necessary, you may desire a more rural lot where you can garden or enjoy peace and privacy. Buy land in exactly the spot that will bring you the most satisfaction.

Determine if you will be living in your home for only a few years, or for decades to come. When at home do you spend most of your time indoors or out? Will you want a garden area? A play area for children? An outdoor spot for exercise or to barbeque? Will this be your retirement home? Might you want an outdoor, yet enclosed swimming pool or open tennis court? How you live will determine the building site you choose, and ultimately the home's design.

Even if you are prone to indoor activities most everyone enjoys looking out a window to see some greenery or local wildlife. Trees, flowers, a vegetable garden, even just a bird feeder or two hanging from eaves offer tranquil additions to a home's environment.

A home should not take up an entire lot. Ensure plenty of outdoor space immediately surrounding the structure. Even if you've opted for a small city lot, don't build edge to edge on it. Leave green space in order to connect with nature on some level, extend a deck or patio, or just ensure breathing space.

One big rule of thumb with a 1/3 acre or more is to never build on the best area or section of land. The reason for this came to me as we walked our 43 acres for an appropriate home site.

If we were to have built on the most obvious open spot with the best views, the rest of the land would have immediately become inferior and of minimal appeal. By not building there, we still have that place – untouched in its natural state. We could set out a garden bench, or pick wild lupines that bloom in early June. We walk there, gaze out, enjoy sunsets and sunrises, and listen to the rhythmic beats of raptors' wings as they pass overhead.

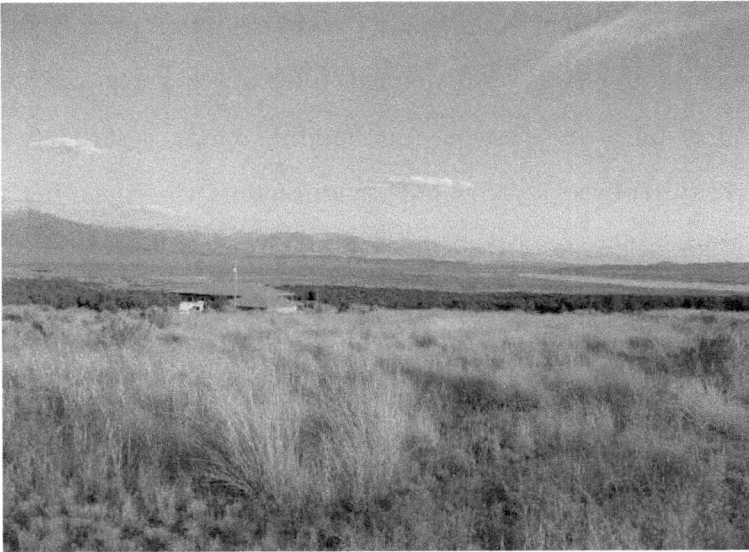

The nicest view spot on the land remains in its raw state. The house still has a grand view and privacy, but we spared this nice spot from disruption.

We opted to put our house just southeast of the best spot. The building site still has outstanding views while maintaining desirable open space. Remember, the quickest way to ruin a place is to inhabit it. Select a site responsibly and build conservatively.

Make sure that usable outdoor spaces offer some level of protection from the elements, afford privacy, or simply support intimate outdoor seating to commune with nature. Outdoor areas should be neither too vastly open nor too shut-in. You don't need solid walls or fences, trees and shrubs can often provide just enough protection or privacy to create a feeling of peace and safety. Too many or excessively tall building wings or garden walls can make outdoor spaces feel like encampments, thus negating any relaxed breezy feeling of the outdoors.

Covenants, Restrictions, and Home Owners' Associations

When selecting a parcel of land ensure appropriate Codes, Covenants, and Restrictions (CC and Rs) regarding what owners can or cannot do with parcels. Subdivision codes can affect what can be built, how a structure appears, and perhaps the materials used. Read the fine print carefully. You may not favor a clause or home owners' association dictating what color a roof can be or that all homes must be English Tudor style with steep 8:12 roof pitches, if your plan was a southwestern adobe style home.

Typical codes, covenants, and restrictions mandate how far a structure must be from property line boundaries, how many structures or residences may be on a parcel, whether or not pets or livestock are allowed, the allowance of non-operable vehicles and so forth.

The opposite of Covenants and Restrictions being too restrictive are CC and Rs that are too loose to maintain property values and neighborhood integrity. You don't want to invest time and money into building a gorgeous, sustainable home that will last for perpetuity only to discover that the person who bought an adjoining parcel decided to establish a huge commercial hog farm or a sea of trailer house rentals.

Home Owners' Associations are similar to CC and Rs in that they also can dictate how properties look and are maintained. Home Owners' Associations may coordinate everyone in the neighborhood chips in to share the cost of plowing or maintaining roads. This can be a great service. Having to pay $3,000 per year for this service may not be a reasonable trade off. Make sure you check, read, and know before you buy.

Water tables and the local ecosystem are everyone's responsibility to preserve and maintain in a healthy sustainable manner, but not all land owners have sustainability or local flora and fauna in mind. A former land owner in our subdivision decided to sell when he heard that domestic water wells produced barely enough water for household and garden use. He had previously resolved to keep several large livestock animals and strip the land of the native Utah Juniper trees to plant feed for the livestock. Doing so would have created erosion, terrible dirt storms when the wind picked up, and drained precious (and fortunately protected) aquifers. He sold after he decided the water tables were inadequate for his "needs".

Keep the above factors as well as any other lifestyle choices that may be important to you in mind as you shop for land or consider the type of residence you want to build. A home's natural and social environments matter immeasurably.

Water and Septic

Water, good water, is critical. Consider the following:

What is the water source for the land or lot you might be considering?

Does every lot or parcel have its own well?

Is there a communal well for an entire subdivision or sections of a subdivision?

Are city water and sewer available?

Is the municipal water system clean and relatively low in chemicals or will it require filtering? Chorine and fluorine may help prevent disease outbreaks, reduce other contaminants, and whiten our teeth, but they are also carcinogens.

If the property is rural you will likely hire a licensed domestic well driller to drill your well, sink a pump, and possibly add a filtration system. If drilling the well drilling company will often provide a choice of either PVC or steel well casing. PVC, besides the residual plastic toxins, can crack with seismic activity. Steel casings can erode slowly via electrolysis. This occurs from the wiring that connects to the submerged pump. Small electrostatic charges, slowly over time, can erode steel casings. Yet, this sometimes never happens and if it does it takes many decades. I would recommend steel for most well situations, but do homework for wells in the area you're considering.

Most wells prove fairly affordable with water easily had in sufficient gallons per minute for household use. However, check local well drilling costs in the area. In our area drillers are in demand for mining exploration, so there are only three licensed domestic well drillers who charge premium prices. Our well ended up being 860 ft. deep. Fortunately, I budgeted for worst case scenarios. Had the well been another 40 feet deeper, we would have had to scale back on the house design to offset well costs.

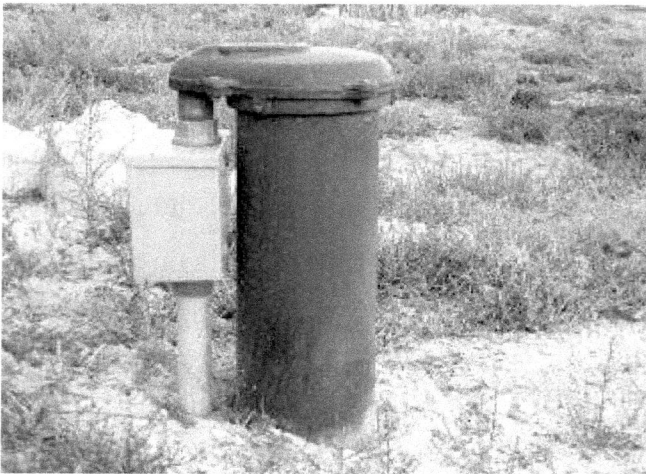

Steel well casing with wiring that travels from the main electrical panel box down to the pump.

Drillers usually charge by the foot. The deeper a well is the more expensive it becomes, and not just due to the depth, but also for the pump and wiring. The more feet of wiring and the larger the pump necessary to pump water from greater depths increases the cost of the well. When metals prices are up, wiring is expensive. The pump and wiring for our well was in excess of $7,000 in addition to the actual drilling cost. Make sure that the cost of your well will not significantly impact project plans.

Drillers often charge for dry drilling. In other words, if they drill and don't hit water they still charge a drilling price per foot, but it's usually less than the cost per foot if water is hit. For example, a driller may charge $30 per foot to establish a functional well, but if he doesn't hit water after drilling for days or weeks, he will charge a dry drilling cost of slightly more than half that amount, say $18 per foot. My directive to our local driller was, "Keep going until you hit." Of course deeper wells require more wiring and sometimes a greater horse power pump, but these costs are minimally consequential as opposed to having no water and still having to pay for the drilling. I recommend, for most situations, the drill-till-you-hit plan.

Don't put any faith in a water witcher or dowser. A witcher is a person who will come out to your building site, charge a couple of hundred dollars, and walk the land either with bent metal rods or willow sticks in hand – divining rods. When the rods cross or veer down towards the ground, allegedly there will be water there and it will be good place to drill. A former neighboring land owner of ours put all his faith in a witcher's advice and ended up with approximately $20K in dry drilling costs. He sold his land at a loss. My brother, who has built two homes, had both his wells witched. In both cases his wells were the deepest and least producing of all the houses in either neighborhood. He's convinced witching does not work. Moreso, there is no scientific basis for witching, hocus pocus might describe it quite well.

Water quality is critical for obvious reasons. Some wells may be bad, and by bad I mean toxic. Veins of arsenic and other unhealthy minerals can be present in domestic wells. Check into wells in the area you plan to build to find out what type of water people have. Phone local well drillers or county offices before you buy. An informed land owner is generally a happier one. If wells seem to be good, have your water tested after the well is drilled. A water test will tell what minerals are in the water and may determine whether or not you need a filtration system. Our water ran, and still runs, heavy with iron and calcium, so we installed a specific iron filter and a softener. Now tap water is super clear and tastes great!

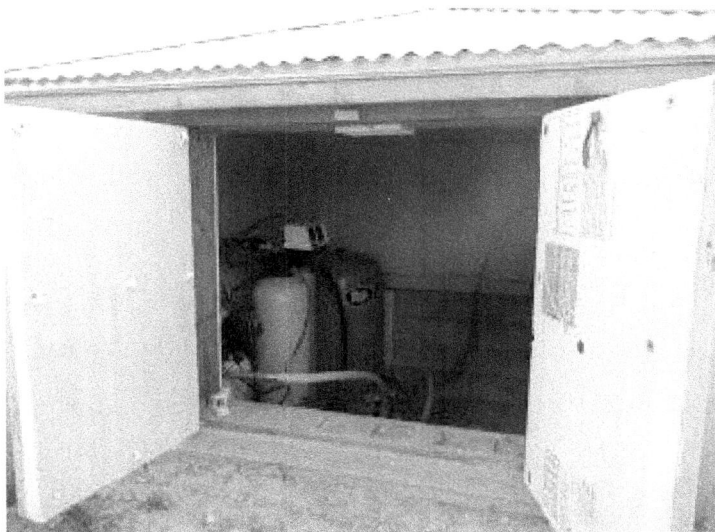

This pump house is well insulated and sheet-rocked. Notice the 2" solid foam on the interior of the doors.

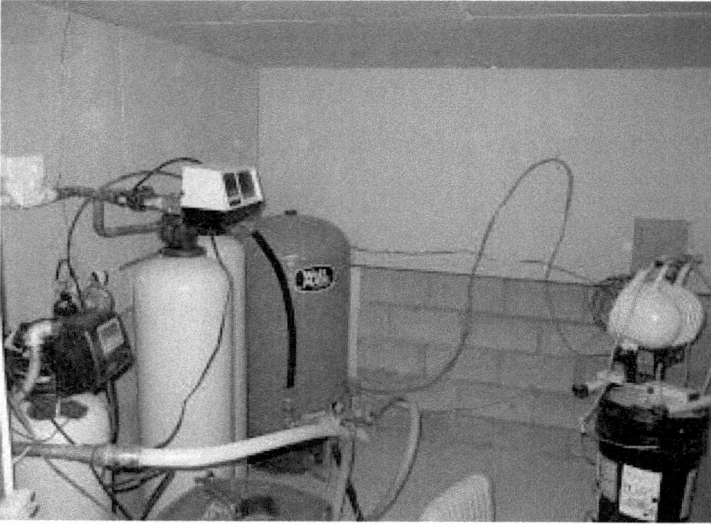

Inside the pump house from rear left to front left: Well Mate pressure tank, iron filter with built in compressor, and water softener.

Rural Septic Systems

Where waste water and storm runoff goes will be another consideration when selecting land and siting the home on the lot. In-town or municipal sewer waste systems are no problem, as you just pay to hook into them. However, if a land parcel is rural it will likely require putting in a septic system. Most often a domestic well and a septic system need to be at least 100 – 200 feet apart for safe drinking water and adequate sanitation concerns – this is usually not a problem. Check local codes for distances in any given jurisdiction or area.

There are several types of septic system designs. The local State Department of Public Health can help determine which type works best for soil conditions on a given site. The Department of Public Health is the office that issues septic system permits after a soil percolation test is done.

In many counties or areas a septic system permit issued by the State Department of Public Health must be in hand to obtain necessary building permits. In some areas the State Department of Public Health will allow you to conduct percolation tests yourself, otherwise you must hire a septic system contractor.

Percolation testing involves digging a small deep trench to document soil stratification several feet down – seven feet is not uncommon. Soil or rock type formations are recorded at different depths in the trench. For instance the topmost foot is likely topsoil, followed by some rock and then clay, sand, or more rock. Sketch the layers and/or take photos so that the State Health Department can see the mineral levels.

The next step in percolation testing requires digging a hole or holes using a post-hole digger and timing how long it takes a certain amount of water to drain from the hole. Typically the holes are about 24" deep and 4" – 12" in diameter. Requirements vary by jurisdiction, but the State Health Dept. will have step-by-step procedural requirements on how to conduct the test.

If you don't feel confident or if local codes don't allow self-done percolation tests, the health department will have a list of people who conduct them in your area. Once the percolation test is completed, an engineer from the State office will put in writing how many feet of drain pipes or percolation is needed. The size will directly relate to the number of bedrooms and bathrooms the house will have. The State office will also let you know what types of septic systems they approve.

Our State Environmental Health office also provides sample schematics of septic system layouts – where a tank must be relative to a structure, how drain lines lay out, and so forth. You can easily sketch this yourself and plan accordingly following some simple and typically legislated guidelines.

It's wise to position a well up hill from the septic drainage system, if possible. Just follow regulations or codes to keep wells and septic systems legal and your family safe.

Sketching a septic schematic is straight forward. You'll show a main, 4", sewer line exiting the home and running to a septic tank. From the tank you will sketch drainage pipes. The tank holds solids, while the lines allow effluent to ease into soil. Pipes must be level, and meet the linear feet required by the state. Lines may run parallel to one another, typically 10 ft. apart, or be a long single row. A smaller area with parallel pipes is more commonly used. I will tell how to dig septic line trenches and put a septic system together in Part II.

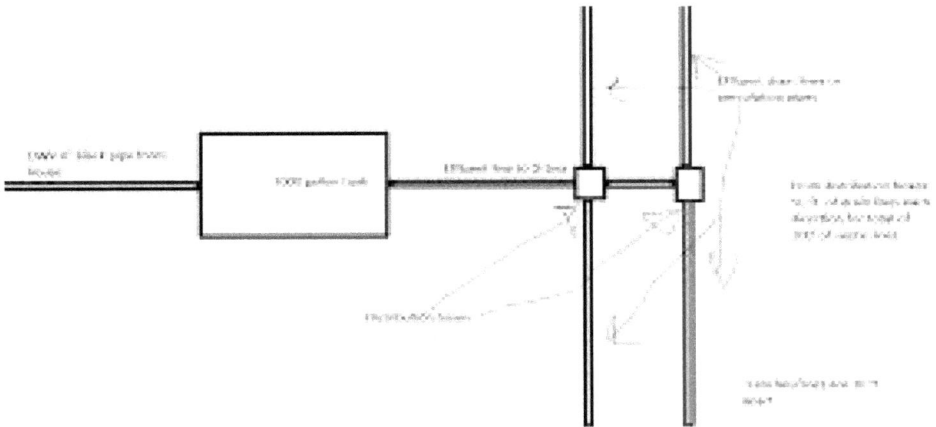

A septic schematic: lines are lower in elevation than the tank.

An alternative to a septic system is having composting toilets combined with a grey water recovery system. There are highly efficient and easy to deal with composting toilets now on the market that work especially well, especially if you have a two story structure with a basement. Sun-Mar, Envirolet, and BioLet are three major manufacturers of composting toilets that have been around for a while and offer some better looking commodes. Some use water, some don't. Some toilets require electricity, but have very low energy draws since composting toilet manufacturers understand that people may be off the grid or use generators.

Composting toilet models that appealed to me were the ones that had smaller, more attractive toilet models with a central composting tank in a basement or lower level to which all the like toilets in the home fed then reduced waste to something similar to ash.

For jurisdictions where kitchen sink water is considered grey water cost comparisons between septic and composting systems are very close. You will not necessarily save money or time installing a composting system over a septic tank and drain field, but you'll be reducing potable water demands.

With composting toilets black water from toilets is taken care of, but you'll need a system to treat or filter grey water - water from showers, sinks, and washing machines, which is still contaminated but less so than sewer waste. Grey water systems can smell just as vile as black water systems and be serious health hazards if they are not installed properly. There are some excellent grey water resources on the Internet and plenty of books available. One book that I purchased on the subject was, Creating an Oasis with Grey Water by Art Ludwig. This slim how-to manual is fairly detailed and can help you get started.

In many jurisdictions kitchen sink waste water is classified as black water. Even with composting toilets a septic system must be installed to process this waste water. Often it's not cost efficient nor environmentally prudent to put in both grey water and septic systems as they both necessitate disturbing natural landscapes, using tanks and pipes, and take time and labor. Weigh potable water savings and installation costs. It may be best to simply install state of the art water saving fixtures like dual flush toilets, waterless urinals, and other low water demand plumbing.

Power

You may opt to build a home that is off-the-grid and uses solar or other means to generate power. Suburban or urban lots certainly have instant and easy access to power, but home owners may opt to combine grid electric with solar generation to save money, reduce green house gas emissions, and make a societal contribution.

Rural locales may require a decision whether or not to run power lines to a home or building site at all. Power companies charge for poles, transformers, and time. Yet, given that off-grid solar with battery backup is still in early adolescence in that the expensive deep cycle batteries have to be replaced approximately every ten years, then perhaps running power to a site is economically and environmentally smarter.

Consider grid electricity's source. Is it primarily generated from coal fired plants? If so, you may definitely want to opt for alternative green energy sources. However, if a home is in the northwestern U.S., northern Nevada, and other areas where hydroelectric supplies most all power needs and you're in an area with fairly low per kilowatt hour rates then opting for grid source power may be a wise, money saving choices.

Compare all options for environmental responsibility and cost savings. Find out how much access to power or generating your own power will cost upfront and overtime, as this can drastically increase the total cost of home construction. I discuss this further in the Active Solar chapter of this book.

In short, think about a household's most basic needs, warmth, comfort, water, and power along with cost to maintain over time. Research what's available in the area and know costs of implementing basic utilities before purchasing land or creating a home design.

Fencing

One lot or land improvement you may want, or have to make before beginning construction, is fencing.

We fenced before beginning construction since we live amongst public land that is leased to a local hobby rancher for open range cattle grazing. We didn't want cattle standing in wet concrete or falling into any possible holes we might dig, since here in the west cattle are still king and we would be financially liable for any harm done to a big bovine. Not to mention that cows rub-up against everything and can do some annoying and costly damage.

You may want to fence to keep small children or animals safe, or simply for privacy.

An alternative to any type of regular fencing is a garden wall, perhaps made out of plastered bales or shrubs which can be very attractive - perhaps Southwestern or Normandy-ish in style. Just remember to get your bales up from direct contact with ground and plaster them well with a coating that will not be damaged by precipitation.

The Future of the Neighborhood

If you plan to live in a home for decades study in which direction the neighborhood appears to be growing. Are improvements or changes in the area in keeping with your vision of a good place to live?

Are any large commercial developments planned nearby that may affect traffic patterns or growth not in keeping with the ideal? Are more and more homes becoming rentals or commercial spaces? Are community centers planned or road improvements?

Try to anticipate what may come or happen in a prospective neighborhood community. Read county or city planning commission minutes as well as recent environmental reports. Find out if there are any environmental impact statements (EIS) pertinent to the area. Often an EIS will have set precedents for number of homes per acre, whether or not ground water can be used for irrigation or small farm purposes, or whether or not deforestation of any sort is tolerated.

It's a good ideas to research real estate market trends. Have land parcels and/or existing homes gradually increased in value over past decades? What draws people to the area? Is there the strong potential for continued growth or residential demand should you decide to sell or move? For some, especially in rural areas, real estate values may be a moot point as they opt for a lifestyle and not so much a grand investment. But, considering that homes are often a middle class person's single largest investment serious time and thought should be applied to any potential area choice.

Green Site Selection

Environmentally and socially responsible site selection encourages creating a home within an existing community, with existing infrastructure, public transportation, within walking distance to community services, and other contemporary municipal services that reduce personal and household use of natural resources and that doesn't disrupt pristine or previously undisturbed land.

Sites within walking or cycling distance to work or school minimize driving or vehicle dependence, reduce green house gas and carbon emissions, and prove good for one's health. Physical activity is good by itself and coupled with the socialization opportunities available within well designed progressive neighborhoods has an added mental health benefit. Talking to people now and again keeps us stimulated and more active; we tend to smile and laugh more.

Choosing land that has been previously developed or disturbed would be good land reuse. Vacant lots amongst other existing houses or infrastructure are also good choices. It's best to leave pristine open spaces untouched.

Sites must reduce storm water runoff via permeable landscaping and driveways. Storm water should not simply flow from roofs onto driveways or landscapes into municipal sewer systems or where it can cause soil and terrain erosion. Ideally storm water should be allowed to soak into soils as if builders weren't present. Green vegetated roofs are good for this, as are well spaced pavers or gravel instead of solid concrete sidewalks or asphalt driveways.

Consider the slope of the natural terrain. Where does or will rain water or snow melt go? Can rain barrels be placed to help with landscape water needs? Is erosion contained? Are oils and other contaminants from vehicles prevented from eventually reaching streams, riparian areas, or other sensitive environments?

Make preserving open space, respecting the natural terrain and vegetation, saving water sources, and guarding ecosystems site priorities. Drive as minimally as possible and try to have easy access to activities you enjoy.

Site Selection Check List

_____Southern Exposure to Support Passive and/or

Active Solar

_____No Flood Zone and Seismically Stable

_____Accessible Roads

_____Access to Public Transportation or Able to

Reduce Driving Distances

_____Covenants and Restrictions – Acceptable

_____Water Sources – Safe, Clean, Good, Well Depths Affordable

_____Power Available

_____Green Space – for outdoor recreation and health

_____Fencing Needed or Not Needed

_____Neighborhood/Area Is Developing in Positive

Ways In Keeping With My Needs/Wants

_____Neighborhood Suits Current and Future Lifestyle Choices

_____Easy to Protect Natural Ecosystems

Chapter 2

Heating and Cooling with Passive Solar Design

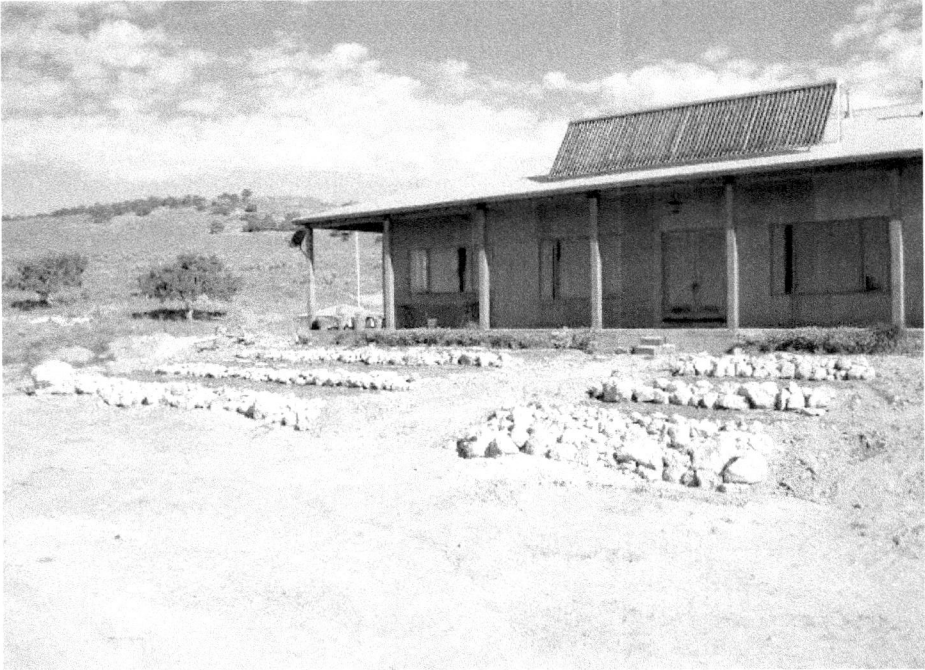

This home is oriented 12 degrees east of true south. Notice that in this June photo no direct sun enters south facing windows

Embedded within design considerations must be a mind toward saving energy and the associated costs. Think of heating and cooling a home the least expensive way possible – passively. Passive solar design means designing a home to use the sun's energy along with local climatic conditions without mechanical systems to effectively heat and cool the home.

Active solar heating means that some mechanical systems such as solar collectors and pumps may be involved. I will discuss active solar for floor radiant heat and domestic hot water in a later chapter.

Depending upon a site's latitude, elevation, and winter temperatures you may need a back-up heat source in addition to passive solar design features. Passive solar combined with an active solar system often is often sufficient to heat and cool a home.

Where we live sub-zero temperatures during winter months are not uncommon. Yet our home stays comfortably warm relying in excess of 90% on passive and active solar heating. We installed on-demand, propane fueled tankless hot water heaters to boost floor radiant or domestic hot water if necessary when or if clouds prevail. We rarely use them. Our 250 gallon propane tank gets filled every three years. This is testament to well-thought passive solar design features and smart active solar system choice. Carefully planning comes back in savings year after year.

The following are each design feature that must be included or considered to effectively implement passive solar design. No one feature works well enough in isolation to amount to much energy savings; each feature works as a matrix with all others.

Orienting a Home on Its Site

June 21st is the longest day of the year in terms of minutes of actual sunlight in the northern hemisphere. This is Summer Solstice. The sun rises early and sets late. On June 21st the sun is highest in the sky, or more directly overhead. Conversely, on December 21st, Winter Solstice, we experience the fewest minutes of sunlight during the day. The sun is lowest in the sky which means the sun traverses a low arc across the southern horizon

These seasonal sun angles mean that if you have more glass on the southern side of your home coupled with adequately deep roof overhangs or eaves, you will get less direct sun in the windows during summer months and more direct sun during the winter; thus, cooler temperatures in the summer and warmer temperatures in the winter for an energy efficient home. No matter what style home you build, it is critical that the longest, most glazed (another word for windows) wall faces as close to true south as possible. The farther off of true south a home's east-west axis lies, the less solar gain it will receive. Aim for less than 15 degrees to either the east or west of true south.

Just because a site is located in a subdivision or neighborhood with existing houses facing the street, doesn't mean your house has to do the same. Neighbors won't be paying your utility bills or living in your home, so orient it on the site that best suits energy-smart requirements and makes the interior environment feel great and function optimally.

Look around prospective building sites. Are there any buildings, trees, or other tall structures that could block light and sun? Make sure that any given site has open southern exposure. Don't assume that you can put solar panels up in any location on the site to garner southern exposure. Solar collectors which are part of active solar mechanical systems are secondary in importance to passive solar design considerations. Design with passive solar as the first priority.

There are two ways to determine a home's orientation - the position the longest wall length faces or how this wall length is situated on the land; one is to use a compass, the other is to use a global positioning system (GPS).

True south is 180 degrees azimuth or circular degrees not magnetic. North and south magnetic poles are not in the same place as geographic poles and also vary over time. The magnetic direction on a compass will be off by approximately15 degrees to the west if facing south.

Once you have established which direction is true south, find or establish a visual landmark in that direction to use a frequent reference point.

Another method of orienting a home's long east-west wall true south is to pound two stakes into the ground that mark long east to west wall that will face south. Tie string between the two stakes, this will suffice for now as the outside edge of a south wall. Stand along the string, as if facing out windows. You should be facing the southern landmark established previously. Slight variations to the east or west may be acceptable depending upon views and whether you want morning light or late afternoon light coming in east or west windows. Use a GPS and walk from east to west and back again along the string line. If the GPS doesn't read directly east or west adjust corner stakes accordingly. This may take a few tries to get it correct.

Not all super energy efficient passive solar homes face directly true south; ours doesn't. Views and site conditions, wanting to block early morning or late afternoon sun, and other factors may necessitate adjusting the long south facing wall slightly.

Our home faces 11° to the east of true south, or about 169° on a circular azimuth compass or GPS. This slight alteration limits mid and late spring sun entering the home, which makes it a bit colder in spring, but disallows hot late afternoon August sun from directly entering west facing windows. Roof eave depth also contributes to limiting any summer sun from entering the home.

If you care to, at this point, establish four corners of your potential home create perpendicular string lines to the first two established east and west stakes. To do this, follow the 3-4-5 rule. On one side or from one corner measure three feet and make a mark this spot with a felt tip pen or other visible marking on the string line. On the opposite side of the corner, measure four feet from the corner and make another mark in the dirt or put in a temporary stake. Measure the distance between marks. If the distance is five feet, the corner is square. If not, adjust temporary stake until a 3-4-5 ratio is exact. Any multiple of 3-4-5 will work, such as 15-20-25 and it's a good idea to always double and triple check measurements to ensure accuracy.

This is Pythagorean's Theorem which is the formula for determining a right triangle or making sure corners are square. Pythagorean's equation is:

$$a^2 + b^2 = c^2$$

In the case of the 3-4-5 rule, a=3, b=4, and c=5.

You will use this quite a bit during the construction process later on as it's a fairly quick and easy method to check for square corners.

When planning a home's site orientation notice other homes in the neighborhood or town. Most often you'll notice that no consideration was given to orientation other than perhaps capturing a view or to be parallel to the fronting street.

In the west's mountainous regions often the best views are either toward the east or west – to view the north-south running ranges. Homes oriented with most of their glass facing east or west become either flooded with early morning light, which causes them to be colder and darker during winter; or in the case of a west facing long glazed wall, overheated with summer's late afternoon sun which often sends the home's residents running to their nearest window covering store to purchase blinds or drapes to keep out blinding and hot sun - thus no view and a much less pleasant living space. A pound of planning saves tons of cures, energy, and logistical headaches later.

Window Size and Placement

For homes in the northern hemisphere there is such a thing as too much glass or over-glazing on the south side of buildings. Residents can be cooked out of main rooms during winter months if there is too much glass for the size of a living space, and also during summer months if there's not enough shade from roof eaves.

Glazed area must be proportionate to total square footage for adequate heat penetration in winter and to keep a house cooler in summer. Proportion and balance is important throughout a home's design, especially for passive heating and cooling.

Early 1970's era passive solar homes used far too much glass and did not sufficiently account for other factors such as eave depths, cross breezes, creating a tight, draft free building envelope, and so forth. The old designs simply were not as outstanding as many at the time thought, though the concept was correct just in its developmental infancy. Now, forty years later we've got passive home design concepts down and highly effective.

On average, the amount of glass or glazing on a south wall of a home should be 7 - 12% of the home's total floor area. Our home's south wall has about 11.5% glazing of the total floor space and this seems ideal. To calculate the square feet of glass, or glazing, your south wall(s) needs, multiply the home's total square footage by .07 (7%) and then again by .12 (12%). This will give you the minimum and maximum square feet of glass your south wall should have.

Homes at higher elevations where winters are colder should have a higher glazing percentage – 12%. Homes in lower elevations and perhaps at latitudes that do not receive bitter winters will require less glazing – closer to 7%.

For example: Total square feet of home: 2,888 located at 41 degrees latitude, 5,800' elevation, cold winters, hot summers. 2,888 x .07 = 202.16 sq. ft.

2,888 x .12 = 346. 56 The 2, 888 sq. ft. home, pictured on the next page, has 250 sq. ft. of glass on the south wall. 11.5% is the amount of glazing for Direct Gain – the term used for this type of passive solar heating.

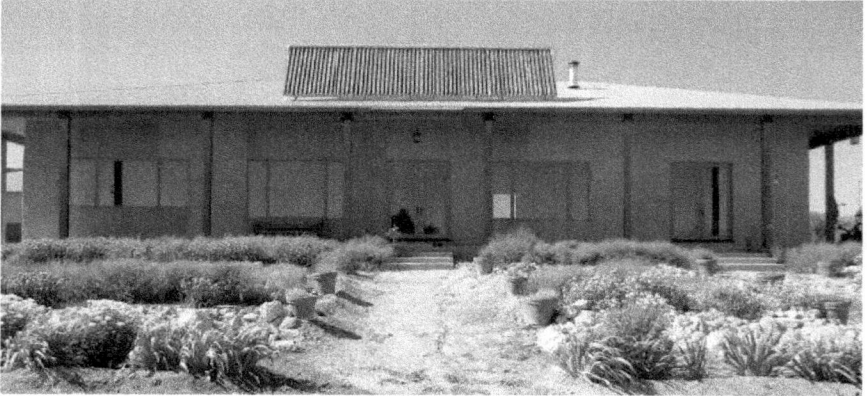

South side of 2,888 sq. ft. home with 11.73% glazing/glass: This amount of glazing also allows for plenty of natural light which saves energy as interior lighting is used less often.

Since the north sides of buildings are generally shaded and colder, it is wise to limit the number of windows here so that less heat is lost during winter. However, do not avoid windows on the north side entirely as you will want breeze pathways that keep the home cooler in summer as well as natural light to make rooms more cheerful and less dependent upon artificial lighting.

If the building site is an area of the western U.S. where late afternoon sun can be sweltering, limit size and numbers of windows on the west side of the home; unless you've oriented your home more towards the southeast where direct western setting sun is minimal.

Early summer mornings are typically cool, so placing windows and bedrooms on the east side of the home may be quite pleasant in that the sun can awaken you naturally, without being too hot, and you will avoid late day or early evening heat so bedrooms remain comfortable.

Roof Overhang

To keep summer sun out of south windows, or east and west for that matter, determine depth of a roof overhang or covered porch. Correct eave or soffit depth blocks summer sun from entering a home, but allows winter sun to bathe and warm rooms. If building a straw bale home, one key principle with straw bale walls is to keep them covered, so a decent roof overhang is imperative for a baled wall home.

Roof Overhangs or Eave Depths

1. Decide upon or estimate the height from the lowest window sill(s) to base of roof soffit. The soffit is the underside of the roof overhang. This is the side you see if standing outside the home and looking straight up to the underside of the roof. If there are any glass doors on the south wall of a home, measure from bottom of doors, or porch height, a few inches either way is minimally consequential. Use the most frequently occurring distance from sill to soffit. For instance if the south side of a potential home consists of primarily glass doors use the base of the door sill as they lower measurement. If there is only one glass door amongst of sea of more highly positioned windows then use the window sill height as this is the predominant glass height.

2. Find your location's latitude, and select the closest cardinal direction that your south wall will face. Choose the appropriate multiplication factor from the chart the follows to determine how much overhang you may need.

If the home will incorporate a porch as our does consider that no porch offers usable space unless it's at least 6' deep. So we have 6' deep porch, which means a 6' roof eave plus the extra foot of roof eave that extends beyond the porch - total soffit depth is 7'. This helps keep a little extra sun off the flat concrete porch in summer. The concrete doesn't heat up and reflect heat back up towards the house.

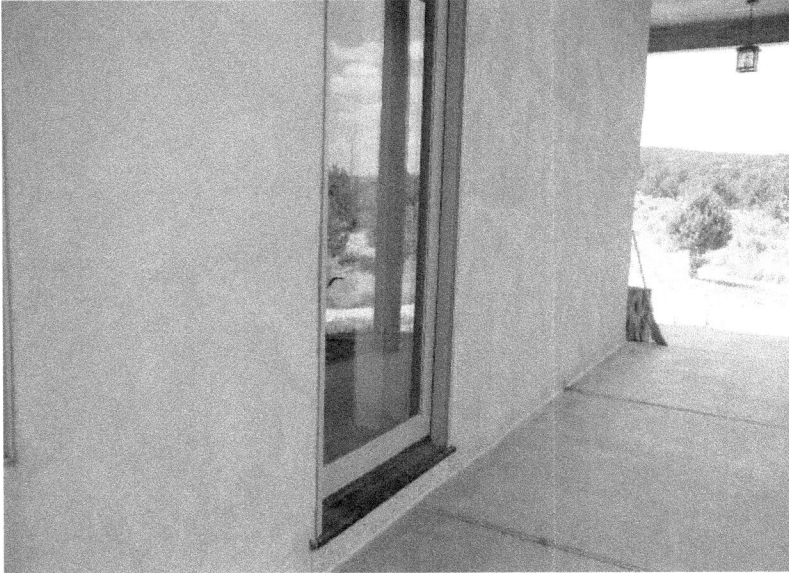

Door sill height of 6" above finished porch height
Sill to soffit height: 12'

Approximate Roof Overhang/Soffit Depths

Calculating solar noon, declinations, and so forth makes calculating roof eave overhangs a bit tricky – this chart provides rough estimates.

	North Latitude (degrees)					
Sill to Soffit Heights (ft)	**35**	**37**	**39**	**41**	**43**	**45**
4'	1'3"	1'5"	1'7"	1'9"	1'11"	2'2"
6'	1'11	2'2"	2'5	2'8"	2'11"	3'3"
8'	2'7"	2'11"	3'3"	3'7"	3'11"	4'3"
10'	3'3"	3'7"	4'4"	4'5"	4'11"	5'4"
12'	3'11"	4'4"	4'10"	5'4"	5'10"	6'5"

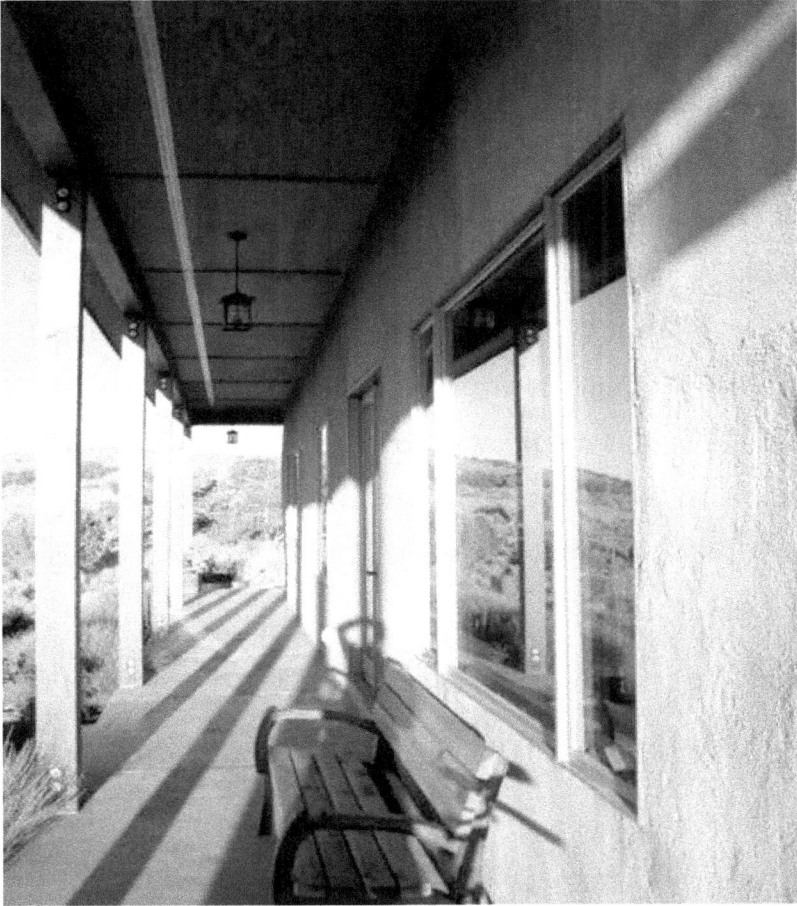

6 ft. deep concrete porch, with 7 ft deep by 12 ft. high soffits

During winter's peak cold months when nighttime lows range from below -10.F to daytime highs in the 30s indoor air temperatures for the home pictured on the previous page are in the mid to high seventies. Most of this warmth is directly attributable to sun entering south windows. The sun radiates into rooms, heats dense tile flooring which retains heat, then radiates this warmth back into rooms after the sun has set.

During bitter sub-zero Fahrenheit winter nights the same home loses about 5 degrees through these same south facing windows since there are no drapes to keep heat in and cold out. Drapes or insulated window coverings kept closed at night reduce heat loss. In this home a wood stove is used to offset heat lost through windows. Wood stoves also add a nice homey ambiance to main rooms.

Wood stoves now have Environmental Protection Agency (EPA) emission ratings. Don't buy one that doesn't have an EPA rating, and make sure you don't buy a stove too small or too large for the space it is intended to warm. Check the BTU output rating, for any stove you have in mind, and the corresponding square footage it is recommended to heat. To keep chimneys as free of creosote build-up as possible stoves must be burned hot. This reduces the risk of chimney fires. If purchasing a stove with BTU output greater than what your area requires you'll not only be uncomfortably hot, but you'll be increasing the risk of a chimney fire as you'll likely rarely have the stove up to higher temperatures.

Wood stoves of course emit carbon into the atmosphere. If you choose a wood stove, use it sparingly and conservatively.

Cord wood is not cheap, nor easily had. We cleared trees off our land in order to build – thus a year's or more supply of wood. Now, we limb trees as part of an ongoing landscaping effort which provides us with more than enough firewood. Think sustainability before installing a wood stove.

Trees

In addition to, or besides eave depth, another way to offer shade in summer and still allow winter sun to flood in your windows, is to plant deciduous trees on the south side of your home. They will leaf out during late spring and summer then lose their leaves to allow sun penetration in winter.

You may not want to use trees if the south side affords a great view. Decide what would work best for your site.

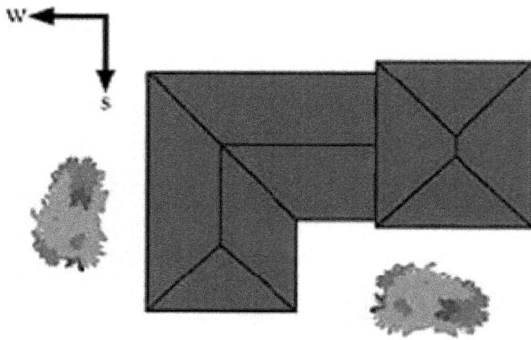

Deciduous trees on the south and west sides of this home in the western U.S. where late afternoon western sun can be sweltering

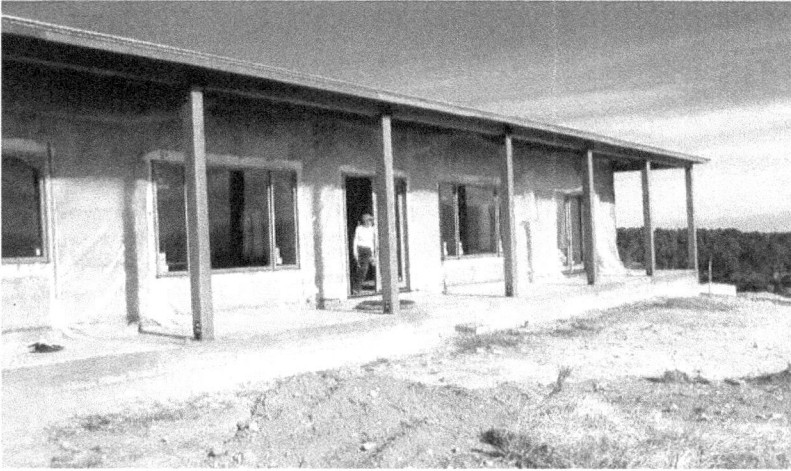

The south wall of a straw bale house: well glazed with correct soffit depths to allow the late autumn sun in. In this photo the author takes a break to look at the views

Thermal Mass

How much warmth is collected within rooms of a home and radiated back during hours of darkness depends upon color and density of flooring and wall materials, otherwise known as thermal mass.

Thermal masses are solid surfaces that absorb, maintain, and radiate heat back into a room long after the sun has set. For example, the floors in the previous example home are ¾" thick Saltillo tile in a terra cotta or medium dark color. Under the tile is ¼" of thin-set, a mortar substance that holds tiles in place. Underneath the thin-set is 4" of concrete, then 6" of sand. Underneath the sand is 2" of rigid foam, and finally a vapor/moisture barrier over a compacted dirt base. This is illustrated below.

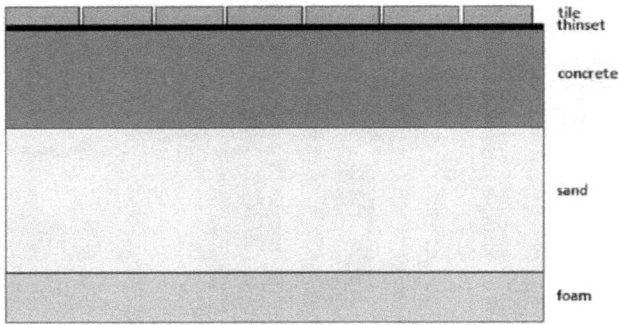

tile
thinset

concrete

sand

foam

A cross section of a home with concrete slab flooring. Floor radiant tubing embedded within the sand is not show.

Sand, concrete, and tile all retain heat. Due to their density, tile and concrete will retain heat more than compacted sand, yet sand allows for floor radiant tubing to expand and contract without risk of cracking. Often floor radiant tubing is embedded in concrete or a more flexible mixture called Gypcrete. This mixture used is not a standard concrete mix but often a product with gypsum added for flexibility to prevent pipes from cracking.

Thermal mass should be uniform in thickness throughout a structure, not concentrated in one area and thinner in another. In other words, don't create a cement slab with tile floors only in isolated areas of the home and use framed subfloors and crawl spaces elsewhere. The home will not absorb or radiate heat evenly or comfortably. The exception to this is multistory homes, where the basement may be concrete subflooring or finished flooring, and upper floors are framed then tiled or finished with some other dense material. Framed foundations or crawl spaces, even with tile flooring, do not create as much thermal mass, or heat retaining qualities as concrete or other hard dense materials. If finished with tile or stone they may have some thermal qualities, but nearly to the extent that a more solid layered subfloor would offer.

Color matters when absorbing and retaining heat. Think what it's like wearing black on a hot day as opposed to white. Make sure floors are of a sufficiently dark hue to absorb the sun's heat, but light enough to minimize dirt showing or other aesthetic concerns.

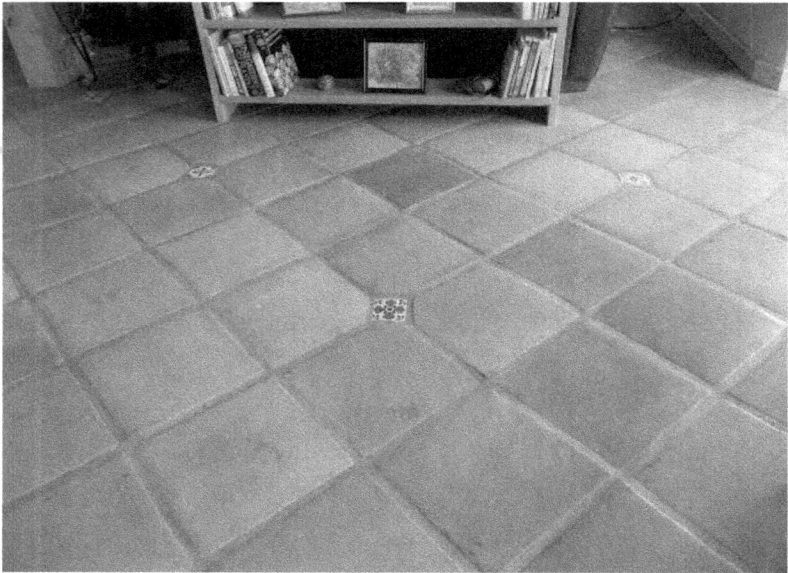

Mexican Saltillo tile, ¾-1" thick of a medium terra cotta color to sufficiently absorb heat

Medium to darker colored walls can also serve to absorb and radiate heat if constructed from dense materials. Before creating dark walls make sure winter sun will actually hit them. Otherwise they will be for decorative purposes only, and dark walls typically make rooms appear smaller.

Breeze Pathways

To keep a home cool in summer create cross ventilation paths via windows that open throughout the home. Generally windows on two sides of every room make people feel better, allow for alternate views, but most importantly provide cross ventilation. With open floor plans you can open windows wide throughout the house at night after the hot summer sun has set, and get cooler nighttime cross breezes flowing. With less open floor plans allow for cross ventilation from windows and through door openings. Know from which direction prevailing winds or breezes blow and plan accordingly.

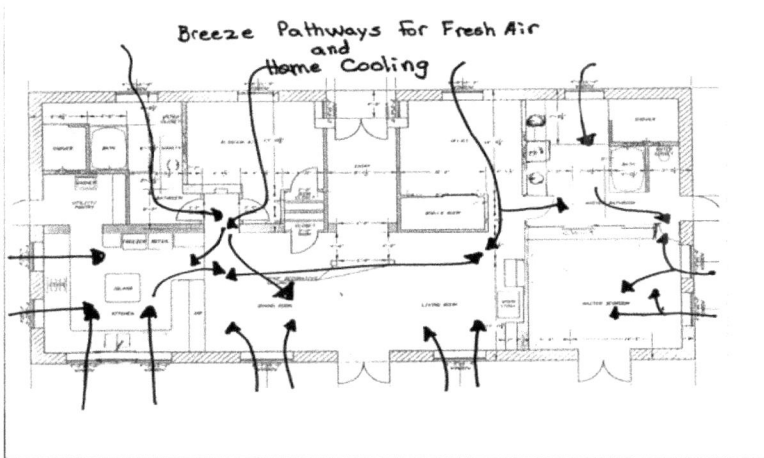

Breeze pathways show where fresh air enters and circulates

Breeze pathways also improve indoor air quality. Numerous studies have shown us that often indoor air is more toxic that what's outside due to household chemical use, off-gassing from formaldehyde containing materials, cooking fumes, inadequately vented stove exhausts, and so forth. Allow fresh outdoor air to circulate regularly during good weather months and occasionally during winter. No one feels good in stuffy rooms and they are not good for us.

High R-Value Attic Insulation

In this age of rising energy costs and inexpensive green insulation there's no excuse not to insulate attic space heavily. A super insulated attic will keep heat in during winter months by not allowing warmth to rise into attic space and out through roof vents to the atmosphere. In summer beefy insulation keeps hot air from permeating down from the attic into living spaces. If using cellulose insulation be aware that it is weighty. Make sure that all finish ceiling materials such as dry wall, wood, or other materials are well attached to bottom truss cords to support the additional weight. Fiber glass insulation is not as heavy but is not a green product. Wool insulation is available, naturally fire resistant, and light weight. It does cost a little more than cellulose.

Make sure that insulation does not cover soffit vents that allow air flow into attic space. Adequate air flow through an attic prevents attics from becoming too hot and reducing the life of shingles or other protective finish roof materials. Air flow through the attic also prevents ice floes, from melting and refreezing snow from destroying gutters or other roof attachments. Attics always must be well vented for roofs to last and homes to stay comfortable.

Reflective Roofing Material

Another factor in keeping a home cool is to select a light color and reflective roofing material so that hot sun is not absorbed into your attic space. If you feel that you must have a medium to dark colored roof, install a solar powered attic fan to exhaust summer heat from the attic and prevent it from migrating down into living space. Check Home Owners Association regulations on roofing, as some areas dictate roof colors and/or materials.

Tight Building Envelope

Make sure all windows are well caulked inside and out upon installation and after, and that doors have good sealing weather stripping. Sealing a home tightly reduces drafts, whether cold or hot, from entering the home, and likewise prevents heat or coolness from escaping. Drafty homes are not comfortable, nor efficient. Don't skimp on quantity and quality of caulk and weather stripping.

Well Insulated Foundation and Sub-floors

Just as attic and wall insulation prove critical, so does an insulated subfloor and foundation stem walls. Breeches of cold air that can reach foundation stem walls and/or crawl spaces cause a home to feel cold. Place rigid insulation up the exterior and/or interior of stem walls; make sure rigid foam is placed under the sand or substrate beneath concrete slab sub-floors. If opting for crawl space or framed subfloors make sure there are no cold air breeches from the crawl space into the home. Insulate subfloor space well, yet do not completely seal off air flow from within a crawl space as this can cause mold, mildew, and dry rot problems.

Other Considerations

Additional passive solar design elements include placing rooms that are most frequently used like the dining room, kitchen, and main gathering spots along the south side of the home. Sunlight will illuminate them naturally during daytime hours thus reducing the amount of non-natural light or energy a home uses. Put less frequently used rooms, such as guest bedrooms, bathrooms, and laundry or utility rooms on the north side of the home.

Open floor plans allow heat to radiate and circulate more broadly throughout the most used areas, like kitchen, dining, living, and office spaces.

If a home has or will have duct work for heating and cooling in the attic or subflooring make sure all ducts are properly tight and sealed with high quality tape to avoid loose fittings and losing heat or cold air into unused spaces.

Attic Fans

In the summer, natural air flow in a well-vented attic moves super-heated air out of the attic, protecting roof shingles and removing moisture.

Attic fans are intended to cool hot attics by drawing in cooler outside air in through soffit vents (soffits and gables) and pushing this air either up through the top of the roof or to channel it through to another side to the outside. Attic fans are now solar operated and inexpensive. They offer a great way to help cool homes during summer. If roof design incorporates a ridge vent, do not install an attic fan. Hip style roofs that have soffit vents typically have ridge vents. Warm air rises up through the soffit vents into the attic area and out the top of the roof. Attic fans would disrupt the natural flow.

I've only discussed direct gain passive solar heating and cooling. There are also indirect gain and isolated gain systems. I do not recommend either for straw bale or any other homes as indirect gain often requires storing heat via walls of water or roof water storage, and the latter involves sunrooms or greenhouse type rooms, both of which contribute to higher humidity or moisture levels leading to molds and mildews.

For more information on passive solar design James Kachadorian has some excellent volumes available, such as **The Passive Solar House**, with very thorough charts that help with design and planning. Also, Daniel Chiras's book, *The Solar House: Passive Heating and Cooling*. Chiras's book may be more readable as Kachadorian's charts and formulas can become complicated for the lay person.

It is imperative to *combine* passive solar design elements. None of the passive solar features work singularly to effectively heat and cool your home. They work in combination as a *matrix* to create a comfortable home environment.

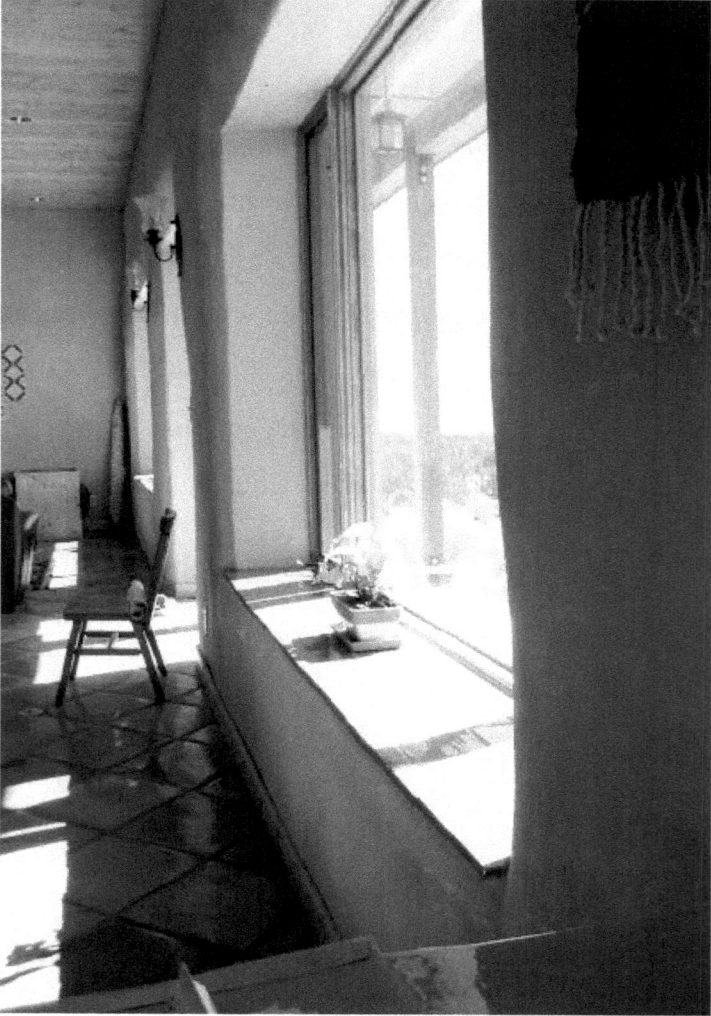

The fall sun warming a main, south facing room, and being absorbed by terra cotta floor and window sill tiles which will radiate heat after the sun has set.

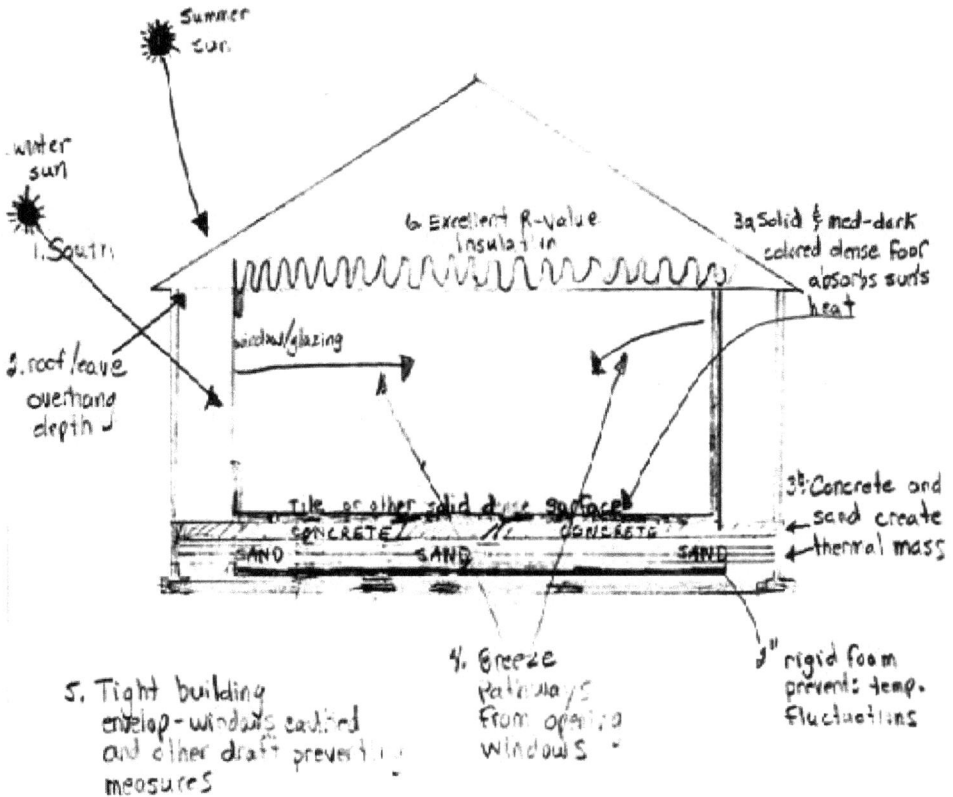

6 Elements of Passive Solar
Heating and Cooling

Summer sun

winter
sun

1. South

6. Excellent R-value
insulation

3a. Solid & med-dark
colored dense floor
absorbs sun's heat

window/glazing

2. roof/eave
overhang
depth

Tile or other solid dense surface

CONCRETE   TILE   CONCRETE

SAND   SAND   SAND

3b. Concrete and
sand create
thermal mass

5. Tight building
envelop - windows caulked
and other draft prevent...
measures

4. Breeze
pathways
from opening
windows

2" rigid foam
prevents temp.
fluctuations

6 Elements of Passive Solar Design:
1. South facing long, well glazed wall; 2. Roof/eave overhang; 3. Solid/dense med-
dark colored floor surfaces; 4. Breeze pathways; 5. Tight building envelop;
6. High R-value attic insulation

Passive Solar Matrix Check List

_____Longest Wall/East-West Axis Faces True South or within 15
   degrees of True South

_____South Wall Glazing is 7-12% of Home's Total
   Square Footage

_____High Quality Low-E, Argon Filled Windows

_____Roof Eave Depth is Correct Ratio for Winter's Maximum
   and Summer's Minimum Solar Gain

_____Floors of Sufficient Thermal Mass and Color

_____Breeze Pathways Through-out Home

_____High R-Value Insulation in Attic

_____Reflective Roofing Material Color

_____Tight Building Envelop – Doors and Windows Well Sealed

_____Insulate Foundation Stem Walls and Beneath Sub-floors

_____Well Ventilated Attic or Attic Fan

Chapter 3

Active Solar Heating Systems

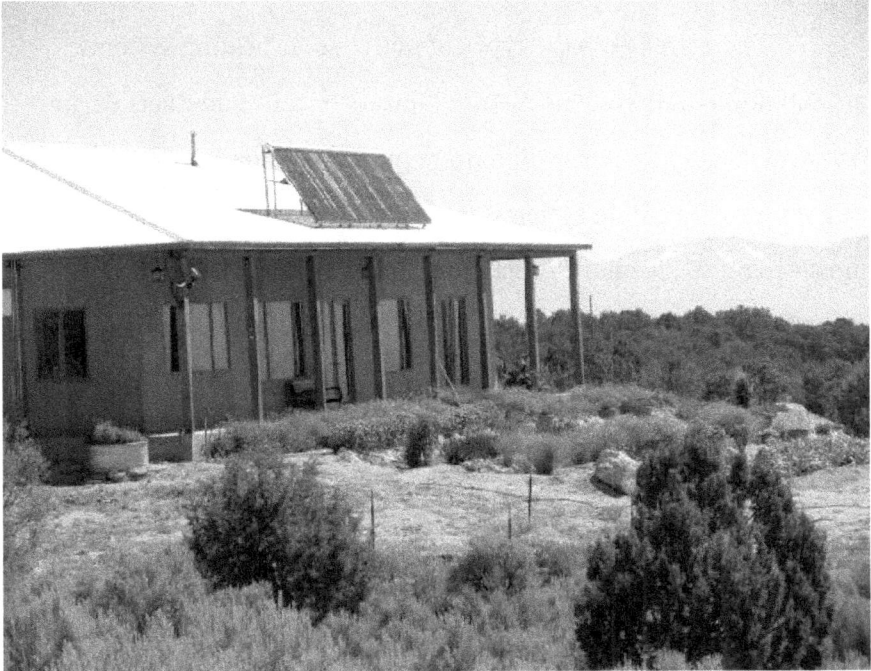

From this distance 64 evacuated tube collectors appear as a flat panel, but are actually 5" in diameter and 5' long individual glass tubes.

Active solar means that there will be solar collectors of some sort, and either pumps to move heated liquid or fans to move heated air. Active systems require energy to run, but in most climates costs much less to install and operate than traditional fossil fuel dependent heating systems. A well-designed passive solar home will require a smaller and less costly heating system of any type, and may need very little supplemental heat other than solar.

There are two basic types of active solar heating systems: air and liquid. Air systems require blowers or fans and ducts or air passages. Liquid systems will require pumps and are best suited for radiant heat. The fluid systems, typically propylene glycol filled, are most often used for floor radiant and other radiant heat sources.

Typically, the solar heated liquid, controlled by a circulating pump, is sent to a storage tank or thermal mass storage to be accessed as needed. Storage tanks, which are most often heat exchangers within a tank housing, store heated liquid that circulates directly into floor loops and that is also used as potable hot water – this is an open system.

Alternatively, heated liquid can circulate within copper pipes inside a heat exchanger tank which is filled with water. The hot copper tubing located inside the bottom of the tank heats water within the tank and additional fluid filled copper coils inside the top of the tank. The fluid in the top coils usually will circulate through radiant floor loops. This is a closed system in that the fluid and water don't mix.

Additional system components include copper pipes, pumps, expansion tanks, gauges, valves, heat exchanger tank, and often a back-up heat source such as an on-demand hot water heater. On demand water heaters only run when necessary, do not store hot water, and are extremely energy efficient.

Choosing an active solar system for a home reduces air pollution and greenhouse gasses by not using as much fossil fuel – from oil, propane, or natural gas.

As an owner-builder, decide how much of an active solar system (or how little) you need. You may want to leave the calculations up to the solar company selling the systems, but if you do, it's best to have a ball park idea of what you need. You don't want someone to oversell you, costing more than necessary. Informed buyers end up more satisfied.

There are many solar system configurations and types. To decide what is best for the home you are designing and constructing, a good place to start might be with price.

Originally we wanted to be off the grid – not run any electric lines to the house – but as I learned more about solar collectors, battery storage, inverters, and the rest of the system components, being off grid didn't seem prudent or cost efficient. Off-grid living is still in its early adolescence; the systems run well enough, but battery storage has not been perfected. Batteries still need to be replaced every 8-15 years depending upon type, and they're not cheap. It's not uncommon to hear of people paying $10,000 and more for batteries. This is a heavy cost once, but every decade begins to negate energy savings. Nevertheless, I had a known national solar supplier provide itemized prices for all components if we were to operate off- grid with battery storage. The total cost for our 2,888 home would have been $47,000 for everything: solar panels, inverters, all components, floor tubing, etc.

I sought prices from the electrical company to run 10 poles to our home site, and for evacuated tube solar collectors to heat domestic hot water and floor radiant heat. The cost for the power was $10,000. The cost for the evacuated tube thermal solar system was $17,000. We decided to go with this set up, running power to the house and garage coupled with solar as our primary heat and hot water source. This is referred to as hydro-solar or thermal solar. Total cost: $27,000; much better than $47,000 for being off grid. We have no batteries to deal with, no inverters, and a much simpler system to install and maintain. At our present annual electricity usage cost of about $40 per month, it would take forty one and a half years before we offset the cost of being off-grid. The bottom line is to shop around, compare systems, and decide what you think will work well for your situation.

Local climate, type and efficiency of collector(s), and collector area all combine to determine how much heat a solar system can provide. It is usually most economical to design an active system to provide 40%–80% of a home's heating needs.

Our floor radiant heat runs daily on sunny and partially sunny days during winter, but it's hard to say exactly what percentage it provides since the home warms up nicely due to its passive solar matrix. Our best guess is that depending upon outdoor winter temperatures and amount of sun or clouds on any given day, our primary heat source is from the passive elements. The active solar floor radiant heat likely accounts for roughly 40% or less during winter.

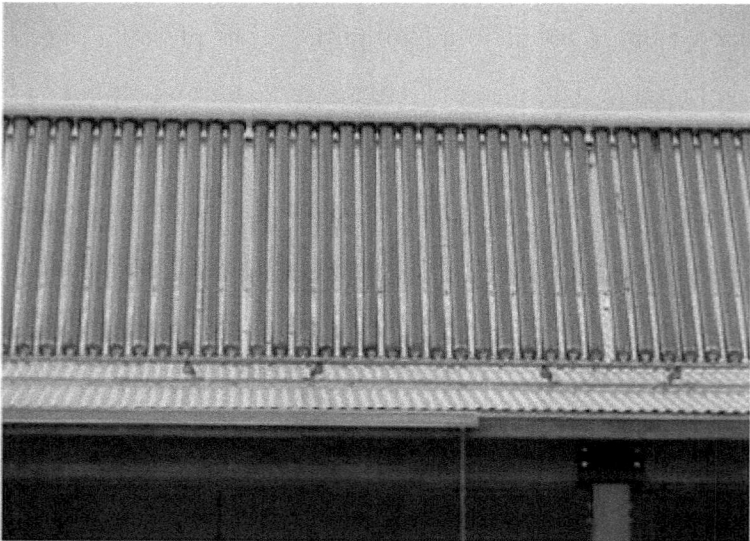

Evacuated tube collectors attached to the header and working well.

Controls for solar heating systems are often more complex than those associated with a conventional heating system because they analyze more signals and control more devices (including a conventional backup heating system). Solar controls use multiple thermostats, switches, and pumps to operate the systems.

Excessive heat or bitter cold can harm solar systems. Sensors, thermostats, and switches are designed to turn pumps on and off automatically when fluid temperatures reach minimum and maximum temperatures. Moving fluids inside the system prevents overheating and freezing. Excess heat is released via copper pipes either underground, exposed to air, or used to heat water – sometimes hot tubs.

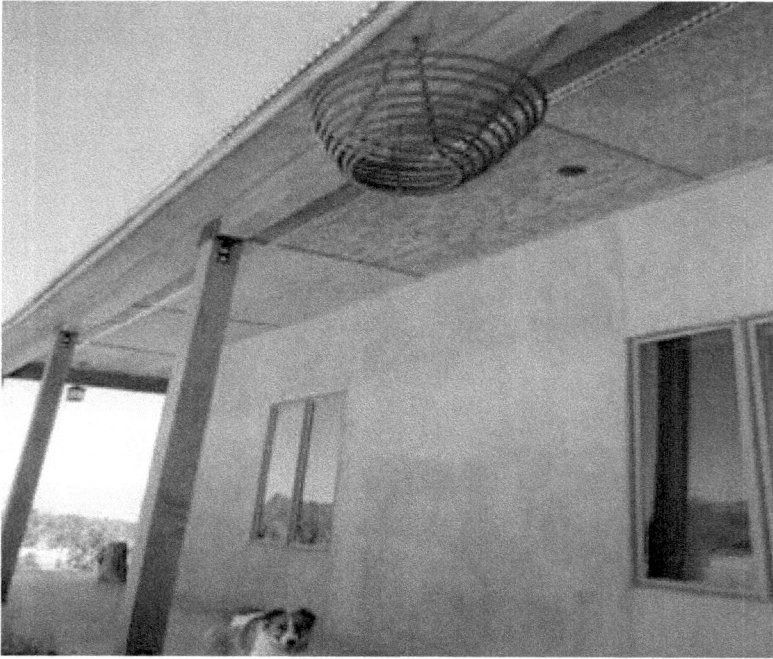

60 ft. of copper tubing exposed to the atmosphere to "dump" excess summer heat.

Mechanical and electronic controls vary in how they operate, perform, and cost. Some control systems monitor temperatures in different parts of a system to help determine how it is operating. More sophisticated systems use microprocessors to control and optimize heat transfer and delivery to a home's heating zones.

When dealing with a solar system supplier know or have at the ready the home's exact floor plan and design. In order to generate accurate bids and system designs suppliers need to know total square footage and where you plan on mounting solar collectors. Collectors may be mounted on the roof or a free standing secure rack. Some fancier racks move to track the sun, but if you have good southern exposure this is not necessary.

The more nearly complete a home design is the more accurate obtaining bids will be. An owner-builder should be pricing materials from the onset of home planning and design to avoid having to cut way back later and redesign because of low estimated costs.

To save money draw floor radiant tubing layouts yourself. This simply means deciding how to run floor radiant tubing underneath the floor. If the home is small one heat zone will be enough. In the 2,888 square foot 2 bedroom home used throughout this book, there are 3 floor radiant zones: master bedroom and bath; main living, kitchen, and library; and guest bedroom, bath, and laundry room. Having three zones, means that a home can be heated where heat is most needed and limiting heat to minimally used areas.

When installing a floor radiant heat system tubing is installed first in the early phases of construction long before flooring is finished and the mechanics of the system are put together. If at this point active solar heating sounds a bit complex for a do-it-yourselfer, don't despair. It's easier than you might think.

Neither Rob nor I had installed a solar heating system before doing so for our home. We bought a system from a Vermont supplier. The floor tubing, pumps, evacuated tube solar collectors, brass and copper fittings, the entire system arrived in several boxes via UPS.

Laying tubing in sand beneath where our concrete slab would be poured was easy and straight forward. We had drafted on a blank floor plan schematic where tubing would run, then placed tubing accordingly, originating and ending each run where the floor manifold would be placed in the mechanical room.

Installing evacuated tube solar collectors on the roof proved just as easy. Rob constructed a stout rack using unistrut metal braces from the local building supply store. He installed the solar tubes' heat collection header along the top of the unistruts, then snapped tubes in place according to directions.

The challenging part came when configuring the copper pipes, pumps, valves, gauges, and electronics in the boiler room. Rob laid the components out on the concrete porch according to how he understood the directions. He then sent photos snapped with his cell phone to the Vermont supplier. Within minutes they phoned him back with explicit directions on what to move where and how to attach component A to component B.

If a mechanical system seems confusing and like us you are not an HVAC or home mechanical professional, simply lay all components out on a large flat surface such as a porch or garage floor, roughly the way directions dictate, snap a photo or two and send this to the supplier. They will guide you through proper placement or layout.

These companies deal with owner-builders all the time and know word of mouth is the best advertising. So snap pictures, call them up, and do what they say. You should be o.k. If all else fails and you just are too insecure with soldering copper pipes or programming thermostatic controls, you can resort to calling a local pro.

Active solar heating will save \money and help establish a home's green footprint. Our home's average monthly electrical and propane costs, as of 2011, were $35.00 and $12.50, respectively. The home has a propane range top in the kitchen and two on demand propane fueled back-up hot water heaters that only kick on when there's inadequate solar gain. All lights, pumps, kitchen oven, and well pump and accessories are electric. With a combination of sound passive solar design and active solar applications a home will be extremely comfortable to inhabit and inexpensive to own.

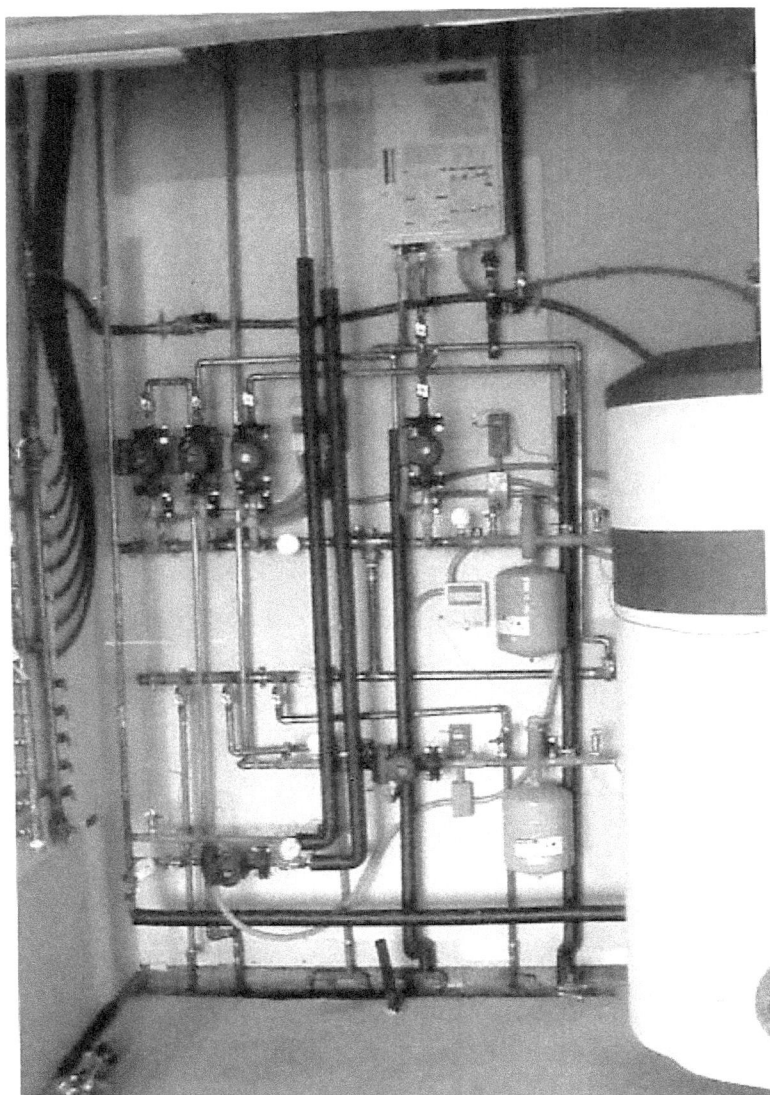

The solar and floor radiant mechanics and electronics may appear complicated, but even do-it-yourselfers can manage accurate and successful installation

Active Solar Check List

_____ Solar Tubes or Panels of Sufficient Size to Meet Hot Water
and Heating Needs (do not undersize a system)

_____System is Cost Efficient to Install and Maintain Over Time

_____Back-Up Heat Source Tied-in to System

_____System Support Easily Available

_____Closed or Open System

_____Floor Radiant Heat Zone Schematics for Optimal
Control and Comfort

Chapter 4

Purposeful Design

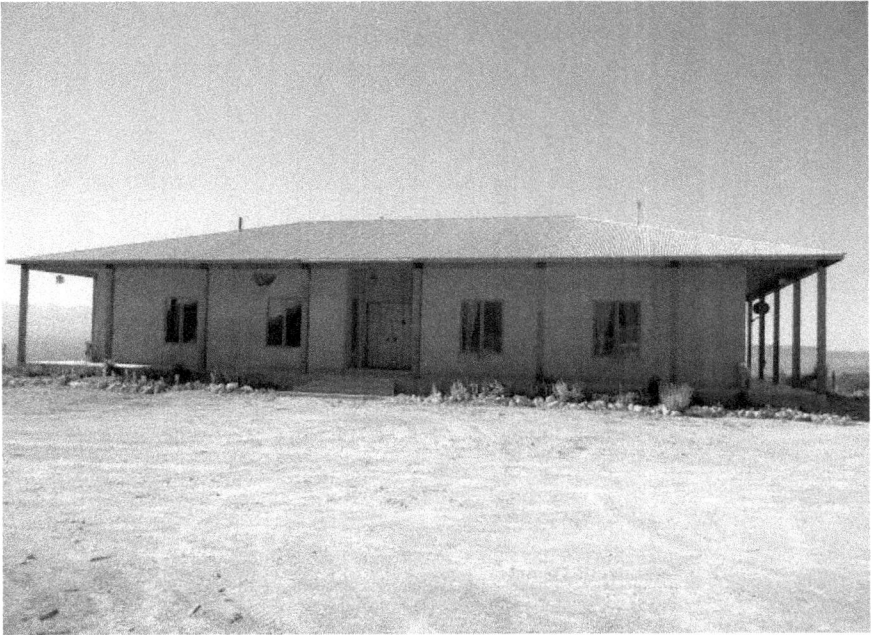

North side of an owner designed and built straw bale home; Notice the essential straw
bale design of up and covered as well as symmetrical window and door placement.

Creating a Green Home

Use green materials and environmentally conscious construction methods when designing and building. The home should be non-toxic to live in, have interior space and exterior landscaping in keeping with what you can afford, have the physical stamina to build, and willingness to maintain. Foremost to keep in mind when designing a home is the structure's quality and longevity. The home should be designed and built to last generations.

Materials used in a home should come from sustainable sources and be responsibly manufactured. You might want to use the U.S. Green Building Council's Leadership in Energy and Environmental Design USGBC LEED) designations as a guide.

LEED for Homes offers great guides with thorough energy and environmental conservation ideas which can be incorporated into the entire design and construction schema. While designing and building I used LEED residential guides, but did not pay for someone to guide us throughout the process or formally certify our home.

Some LEED (and sound) Residential Construction Considerations:

• Home is above a 100 year floodplain

• Do not build on habitat that is threatened or where there may be endangered species

• Do not build within 100' of water

• Control erosion as much as possible

• Minimize the area disturbed during construction (In our area lightning strike fires happen regularly, so the U.S. Forest Service recommends 100 ft. of defensible space around a home – we did this even though it is not in keeping with LEED.)

• Be within walking or cycling distance to community services

• Reuse water

• High efficiency irrigation system

• High efficiency plumbing and electrical fixtures and fittings

• Design, mechanical systems, and appliances for exceptional energy efficiency

• Framing practices reduce waste (This is where good planning and math skills come in.)

• Use Forest Stewardship Council (FSC) certified lumber

• Construction and interior materials reduce or eliminate off gassing of toxic gasses, e.g. formaldehyde

• High R-value and green product insulation

• Exceptional quality windows:

• Low E, argon filled, double pane

• Air infiltration and heat loss should be minimal

• Use of renewable energy systems

• Materials sourced from nearby or relatively nearby manufacturers

Making your new or existing home green means respecting the environment through prudent energy use, landscaping, and construction methods and using non-toxic products in your home, or at least keeping them to a bare minimum.

Toxic materials can include: vinyl clad windows, spray foam sealants, compressed and rigid foams, adhesives, oil based paints, stains, and sealants, vinyl flooring, Formica - Formica itself isn't toxic, it is a hard plastic, but it is usually mounted on particleboard backing. Particleboard emits a lot of formaldehyde gas which is a volatile organic chemical. Volatile organic compounds or chemicals are toxic. You may have heard of this as off gassing. Off gassing occurs when materials emit harmful vapors into the environment. Many modern wall-to-wall carpets and area rugs also emit VOCs which have been known to cause headaches, nausea, and other maladies.

Less than ethical marketers sometimes try to attach a green label or claim to products to increase sales. This is referred to as "green washing" when marketers or manufacturers claim a product has green qualities that it doesn't or claim that a product has more than it actually does. Be leery since the construction industry is one of the worst for making these claims.

Some green products worth serious consideration when building or remodeling are:

• Eco-friendly flooring – bamboo, cork, Forest Stewardship Council certified hard woods, clay based tiles, etc.

• Eco-friendly paints and wall surfaces

• American clay, Green Planet clay paints, Fresh Air from Home Depot, and others -Forest Stewardship Council certified lumber, harvested from and by companies that use sustainable forest practices

• Natural fiber carpets, rugs, drapes, and other furnishings – organic cotton, naturally dyed wools, jute, sisal, hemp, etc.

• Recycled glass tiles – these can be used for counter tops or other applications

• Recycled glass, cork or other materials for counter tops

• Green Fiber – cellulose insulation

• Aluminum-clad wood frame windows with the Forest Stewardship Council (FSC) certification, or Sustainable Forest

• Initiative label include: Sierra Pacific, Loewen, and Marvin.

- Eco-friendly cabinetry, counter tops, and millwork.

- Products easily had locally and not shipped great distances

- Environmentally and family safe cleaning products

Concrete and steel have proven fabulous construction materials – strong and durable. However, steel takes enormous amounts of energy to manufacture and iron ore, steel's raw material, is mined. There's no jury still out on mining's environmental costs. Mining is an environmental nightmare, but due to better environmental engineering and E.P.A. oversight it's slowly coming out of the dark ages.

Local building inspectors will likely require steel in foundation other areas of construction, but you don't have to go overboard. The combination of steel and concrete makes for extremely permanent and durable structures that withstand seismic activity such as earthquakes and limit damage due to settling.

Concrete's primary negative environmental impact is the considerable emission of greenhouse gases, such as CO_2, when producing Portland cement. 1 ton cement produces 1 ton CO_2 and other greenhouse gases. There are new "green" concretes on the market such as concretes that use recycled materials in their base and concretes made using fly ash or silica fume in the mix design in place of Portland cement.

Fly ash, the byproduct of coal fired power plants can contain heavy metals such as arsenic, lead, and mercury. Not only is it not green it's deadly.

Silica fume is a byproduct of producing silicon metal and ferrosilicon alloys. It's relatively safe, can have very high strength ratings and be considerably durable. Silica is considered a nuisance dust and like with all concrete, mortar, and plaster mixing requires wearing a dust mask. Avoid breathing in the fine dust particles.

Greening a home isn't a simple one step move. Like a successful passive solar design matrix, making a green home means utilizing as many healthy and environmentally conscience options as possible. Your home may not be 100% "green". Ours certainly isn't, but owner-builders can make their homes much healthier and more economically and environmentally sustainable than most homes currently out there.

Three critical areas to NOT scrimp on quality materials or the time they take to build or install are: foundation, windows, and roof. High quality concrete, steel, glass, and roofing materials are worth every dime a supplier charges. Nevertheless shop around for best bargains on top quality products and take time to install them properly.

Purpose First, Art Second

Make a short list of what domestic, in-house activities matter most, then design rooms and spaces for what you love and the life you live. If you read voraciously - make a library. If you enjoy cooking create a kitchen that suits your cooking style. Whatever you or other inhabitants enjoy, make sure the house accommodates those who will live there.

Ask other inhabitants, like your spouse, to list two or three rooms or at home activities that are important to them. Often family members' wants and needs overlap. Consider a large office space for two desks, or perhaps a kitchen big enough for two, three, or more people to prepare food simultaneously.

To make a house truly great follow one critical rule throughout: ensure that *form follows function*. In other words think of the purpose and use of spaces first, then allow the design to suit the purposes, otherwise you'll have a home that doesn't feel right or work well. Designing rooms to suit your needs and movements naturally makes them work well and feel good to inhabit. Envision yourself walking through the home doing daily tasks. Plan and design according to human movements and habits.

After considering purposes and how you and your family moves and functions within a home, think of how you want useful spaces to appear. This is where taste and artfulness come into play. Walls, their placement, thickness, height, appearance, color, and purpose radiate the home's personality.

Straw bale walled homes feel solid and safe - what walls of a home ought to be. They are not rigid, angular, stiff in appearance, or perfectly straight like common gypsum board walls. Bale walls offer character and a story into living spaces. They are warm, inviting, and homey. Given this, you may consider that interior walls also be made of straw or at least fake the appearance by offering a thickened look.

Size and Shape

Decide upon a single story or multi-level home. Study architectural styles that appeal to you. You may already have a vision of how ornate or minimalist you'd like the home's exterior and interior finishes to look. These determinations will affect construction costs, time, and ultimately the feel of the space you inhabit.

We've all seen or lived in common generic tract homes or apartments that show very little attention to detail and have zero nice finish materials or craftsmanship. Often builders and owners get caught up in size and forget about quality. You will want a house that ultimately satisfies you in qualitative ways such as comfort, design, nice details, and quality finish work, rather than quantitative ways that simply reflect vast square footage, number of bedrooms, or how many stories.

I find the question, "How big?" silly as it poses no interest in how structurally sound a home is or how stunning the finish work. Huge homes do not necessarily reflect quality, nor are they necessarily comfortable to live in.

One of the most beautiful homes I've seen was a small one bedroom cabin-type home in western Montana. The owner-builder took a couple of years to build it with arched exterior beams, hand hewn 16" diameter log posts, and exterior window trim wood work that was flawless. The home reminded me of a forest cottage in a fairy tale; stout and nestled on the land – meant to last and be beautiful for a couple of lifetimes at least, and it was no larger than 1500 square feet.

Tract homes in the U.S. are built purposefully to last about twenty years. The reason for their existence is to fill market demands for various levels of affordable housing, one that in the past and still, offers little regard to energy efficiency or artisan craftsmanship. They also serve to contribute to capitalistic ideals of convincing and actually forcing consumers to purchase more and more. Tract homes, put up by crews as quickly as possible, to satisfy local markets have reduced quality construction, use less interesting materials, and are designed and built to be replaced. Developers' goals are to maximize profits not establish a lasting legacy of quality construction.

I feel badly for more wealthy home owners when I walk into high end tract homes that cost a half million dollars or more, have marble or granite counter tops, decent fixtures, acceptable but not ergonomic floor plans, and see that craftsmanship throughout the building processes obviously lacked. Thus, owners find themselves replacing this or that within a year or two.

The average tract home was meant to be completely replaced: roof, parts of the foundation, mechanical systems, framing (if there's dry rot or other deteriorating factors) every fifteen to twenty-five years. This is hardly a lifetime, far from sustainable, and not even close to leaving a legacy of quality architecture to future generations.

Craft a home that's beautifully finished. Reserve approximately 10-15% of construction budget for finish materials. Finish materials include trim around doors and windows, fixtures, appliances, flooring, counter tops, anything that is visible when the home is complete.

Multiple story homes, especially ones that utilize a basement as either garage or living space, save money. More concrete is demanded for a daylight basement or garage-basement with living space above it, but the basement is utilitarian space.

With multi-story homed there are smaller footprints or foundation areas, thus using less concrete and disturbing less ground. The roof areas will be smaller as well since there will be one roof over two or more levels of home. Simply put, multi-story homes reduce foundation and roofing costs as compared to the same square footage on one level.

If you are middle-age or older and want to stay in your home for as long as physically able, consider a single story home. A single story home allows for the possible eventuality of having difficulty ascending or descending stairs, or using a wheel chair or walker. We considered this and designed accordingly creating 3' wide door openings, wider walk-in shower entries and the like in the event either one of us becomes less able, or rather, when we become less able.

Regardless of age, health, or mobility issues like wheelchair accommodations, larger spaces feel better. Large doorways make moving furniture easier. Large showers make showering more enjoyable – two can shower at the same time which feels like and is such luxury and decadence.

Consider plumbing outdoor showers. Using outdoor showers during good weather not only feels to the body and soul fantastic, but outdoor showers cut down on the amount of moisture in a home and the amount of energy used to operate bathroom exhaust fans. Just make sure to disconnect and drain exterior showers for winter so fittings or pipes don't freeze.

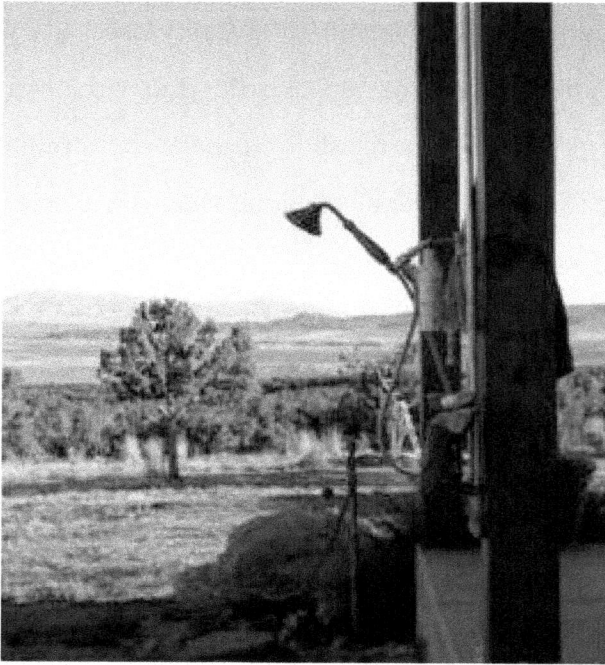

A small, easy to install luxury – an outdoor shower with a grand view and total privacy.

If you have a young family you may want children's areas of the home where they can play, store toys, and read books. Parents will need spaces near the children's area that allow privacy to work, yet allow easy supervision and quick access to the children, or them to you.

Proportions and symmetry affect human perceptions of beauty. People are drawn to balance as well as proportioned asymmetrical forms. As you view photos of homes' interior and exterior spaces look for symmetrical shapes and forms which contribute to serenity outside and in. Balanced asymmetry offers the same affect. Think scale and proportion in all aspects of design. I cannot stress this design aspect enough. Balance every detail.

Begin looking at specific details of attractive homes. What is it that makes the home appealing? Is it a combination of design elements and materials? Is it the setting? Roof slope? Materials? Make a list of all you find attractive.

Why do some windows invite us to gaze out while others simply allow in light? What is a good height for windows where a view is important? If a person is seated can they still see out windows?

Perhaps windows should be no higher than 24" from the floor, or lower in areas where snow or animals can't brush against them. Maybe in tightly built neighborhoods window sill heights need to be higher to afford privacy and safety? Window placement is paramount for an overall good design. Take time and care in planning windows.

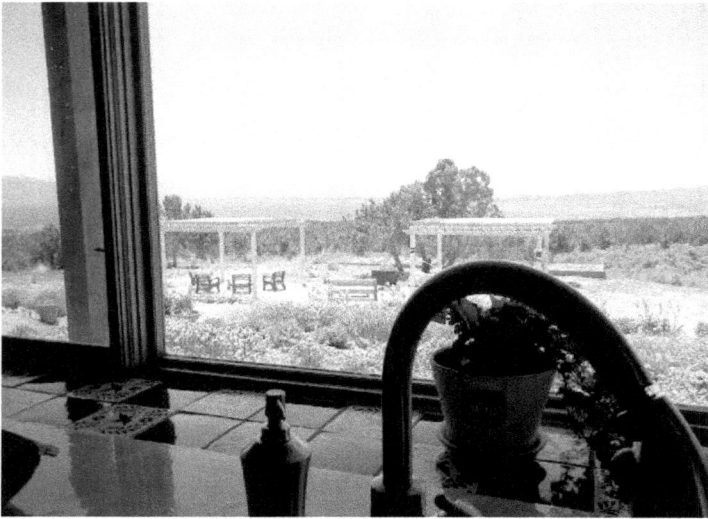

A well planned window allows whoever is washing the dishes or preparing food to observe the natural world.

If entertaining large groups on a regular basis you may want a big kitchen and dining area as well as an outdoor patio space for outdoor hosting.

Make lists of what you want to include or have in your home and design appropriately. Check the list frequently as your sketches change to make sure you don't eliminate something important to you.

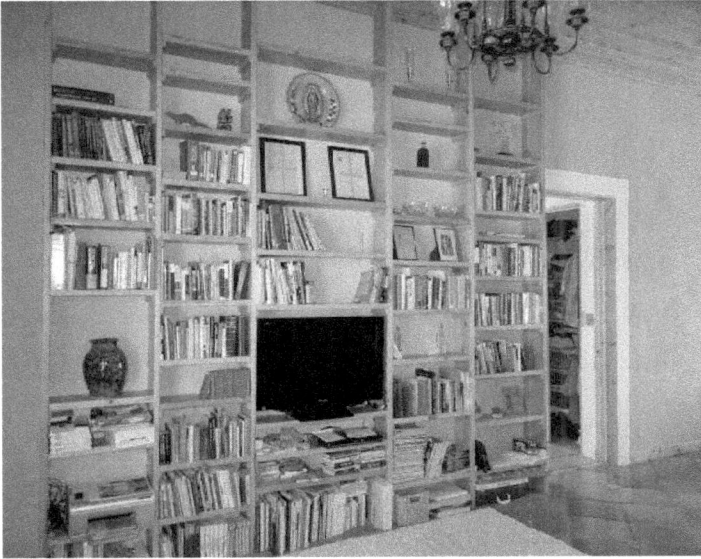

A library room was important to us, so we simply created a room with plenty of bookshelves and a small media office center.

Once basic floor plan sketches are more or less satisfactory, allow a lot of time and thought for determining lighting. Ensure \ambient, task, and area lighting in each room. Do not put switches behind doors where they are difficult to access.

Think through thoroughly every small detail of a home's function and design. Careful planning saves living with years of annoying design flaws.

Conserving Materials and Lowering Costs

Give serious consideration to structural framing members. Decide upon ceiling height(s), framed wall thicknesses, and overall lumber or materials use and cost. To save money use standard lumber dimensions.

Think: conservation. Reuse lumber. Minimize waste.

Lumber comes in standard lengths. Most boards used for framing are called "two bys". This term refers to boards that are 2" (actually 1 1/2") by another dimension in increments of 2" (actual dimensions are always slightly smaller). There are 2 x 4s, 2 x 6s, 2 x 8s, and so on. These boards come in lengths of 8', 10', 12' and so forth, in 2' increments.

Avoid odd numbered measurements for wall lengths and ceiling heights. 9' ceilings require cutting 1' off 10' boards. 9' ceilings also mean cutting drywall and other materials that come in standard even numbered dimensions. Creating a home with nonstandard dimensions wastes countless resources.

If you decide upon 10' ceilings, order10' boards; any longer and you will be wasting and paying unnecessarily for lumber. Finished ceiling height will not measure precisely 10', but it will be very close.

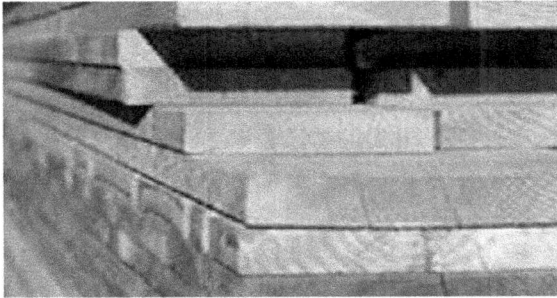

2x6s on top of 2x10s, neatly stacked

Posts and beams offer a stouter feel and are in fact stouter lumber than 2 bys. Common post widths are 4"x 4", 4"x 6", 6"x 6" and so forth and come in standard lumber lengths.

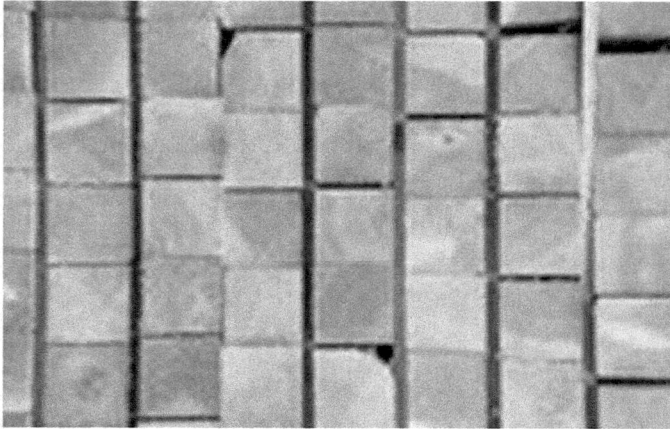

4x4 lumber – a common use is posts

We opted to use 8"x 8"x 12' posts instead of 6" x 6" x 12' posts originally delineated in blue prints. Stylistically, the 6"x 6"s offered a less stout appearance though structurally they were fine. Going larger is not typically an engineering issue for vertical members (use common sense here or check with an engineer if you are unsure) going smaller is. If we had used 4" x 4' posts, we would have needed more of them at different spacing intervals which would have required engineers and the local building inspector's involvement, as well as altering the aesthetics of the exterior.

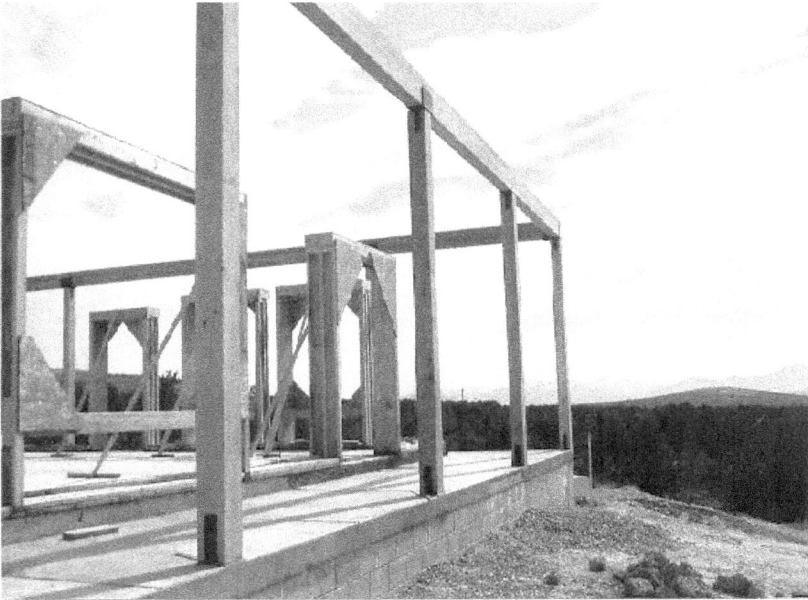

8"x 8"x 12' posts topped by 6"x 12"x 25' glue-lam beams work together as an exoskeleton post and beam design; inside the post and beams are interior window and door bucks. Do not use glue-lams for interior spaces unless you know they are formaldehyde, or other toxic glues, free.

Solid beams are available in the dimensions noted above for posts. However, engineered beams are often used for horizontal applications. Engineered beams, commonly called glu-lams, are more cost effective and structurally sound, but less environmentally friendly due to adhesives used to bind them together.

We used 6" x 12"x 25' glue-lams for a post and beam exoskeleton; which means that planks of 2"x 6" lumber were laminated together for a thickness of 12"w and 25' l. Using solid single planks of lumber in longer lengths risks accepting splits, cracks, and knots that may weaken beam integrity. Engineered lumber is super strong, but check for toxicity before using it in interior spaces.

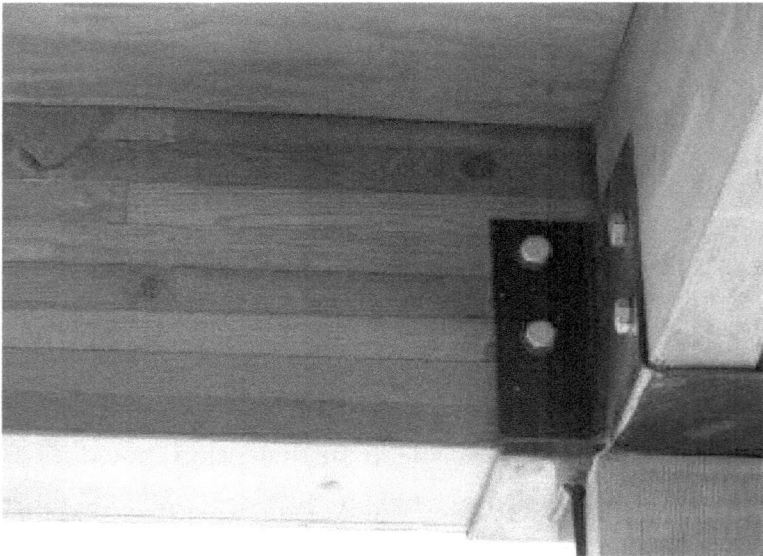

A 6"x12" glue lam adjoined at post corner by a Simpson bracket

Engineered lumber often offers greater structural integrity, and may have a greener nature than Forest Stewardship Council certified single dimension boards. Smaller trees can be used to make engineered lumber, thus leaving larger older growth hardwoods untouched.

Straws Bales

Straw bales come in various sizes depending upon baling equipment. Before determining final wall dimensions, telephone suppliers to find out what dimensions bales might be. This information is critical to have when determining wall lengths and widths. Don't design an entire home to scale only to find out that you can't get the bale size planned for.

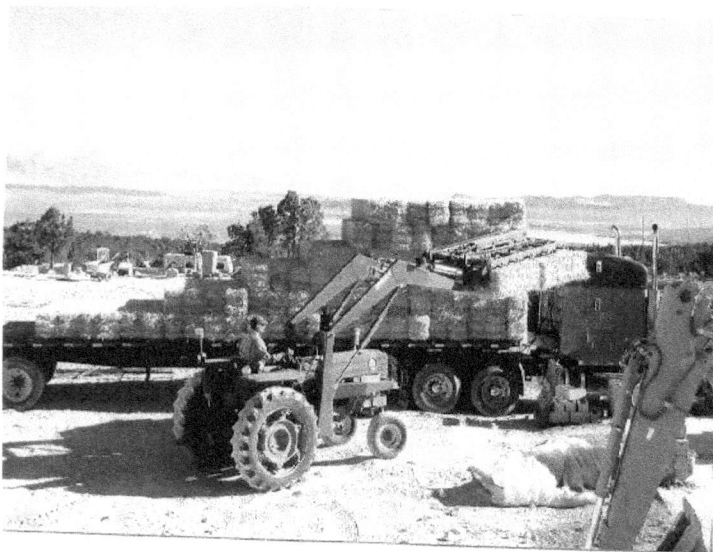

Straw bales being delivered and unloaded. Each bale was checked with a moisture meter in three places - near both ends and center to ensure dryness – less than 12% moisture reading. Ultimately the bales averaged around 6% moisture – ambient humidity for the high desert.

Homes that have more than one roof angle, more wall corners, more wings, and varying shapes in their structural design cost more. A general rule of thumb is that for every corner, beyond the basic four for a rectangle or square, add 3% to the building cost. This is true even if you don't hire labor.

Your time is important, so to complete a home's design and construction in a timely manner keep in mind that the more angles and corners the more thought and engineering during every phase. During construction, corners and angles take more math calculations, more cutting of lumber, more time to create - from the foundation to finish.

Odd numbered and nonstandard wall lengths and heights mean more splitting and retying of bales. There's a reason why so many straw bale homes have simple foundation layouts and roof lines. They are easier for do-it-yourselfers to build and cost less in materials and time.

If your heart is set on a round building don't despair, just be prepared for the increased bale trimming, wood cutting, and so forth. Careful calculations, planning, and fine carpentry skills can make round homes somewhat easier, but not as easy as structures that utilize standard even numbered lumber dimensions, and 90 or 45 degree angles, or corners.

In round homes or in homes with rounded features, determine arcs to cut roof sheathing and other materials with curved edges. Anytime a rectangular piece of wood such as plywood or roof sheathing is cut to create a curved edge, the cut edge of the material often becomes scrap. Careful planning may allow using cut away pieces other purposes – think carefully and take time planning.

Do not burn pressure treated lumber in a wood stove or elsewhere. Pressure treated lumber, plywood, oriented strand board (OSB), and glue-lams contain toxic chemicals that cannot be burned in a wood stove or fireplace. Treated lumber should not be used for interior construction. Treated wood products are for exterior use only unless specifically manufactured safely and boldly designated for interior use.

When drafting floor plans, minimize plumbing and electrical materials by using shared plumbed walls and not running plumbing through walls unnecessarily. In other words, place kitchen and laundry room plumbed walls back to back, or have the laundry room and a bathroom share a common wall. If the home is 2 stories or has a usable basement, design so that plumbed rooms are atop one another so pipes share a common vertical wall.

Avoid plumbing straw bale walls altogether. It can be done by running PEX or other pipes in chases which are enclosed larger pipes to protect bales, but why go to the trouble of channeling out bale walls and the expense and unnecessary resource use of buying conduit or pipes to encase water lines. Remember to keep this as simple as possible. The home will feel better, be cheaper to build and operate, and more comfortable to live in

Load Bearing Walls in Straw Bale Homes

A load bearing wall is a wall that helps support roof and/ or upstairs weight. Load bearing straw bale walls are primarily peripheral exterior walls, but sometimes include interior walls. Roof or upper story loads bear on top of the straw bale top plate which transfers the weight through the bales down to the foundation.

Tests show that the plaster skins, stucco or lime plaster, on both sides of the bale wall will be enough to offer rigidity, or shear strength, to support the walls. Lumber is still needed for window and door bucks, as bales cannot be supported by window frames, nor can window frames be supported solely by straw bales.

In a post and beam structure loads bear on beams with weight transferred down posts and ultimately to foundation footings.

If simply framing a home using common framing techniques and styles and using straw bales as infill, the roof load will bear on the framing members, typically plywood sheathed 2" x 6"s, referred to as modified posts and beams.

If a home is small or moderate in size interior walls that support roof loads are likely unnecessary.

In larger homes, depending upon size and style, interior framed walls may be needed to help support roof loads. Engineers who finalize designs into blue prints will determine this.

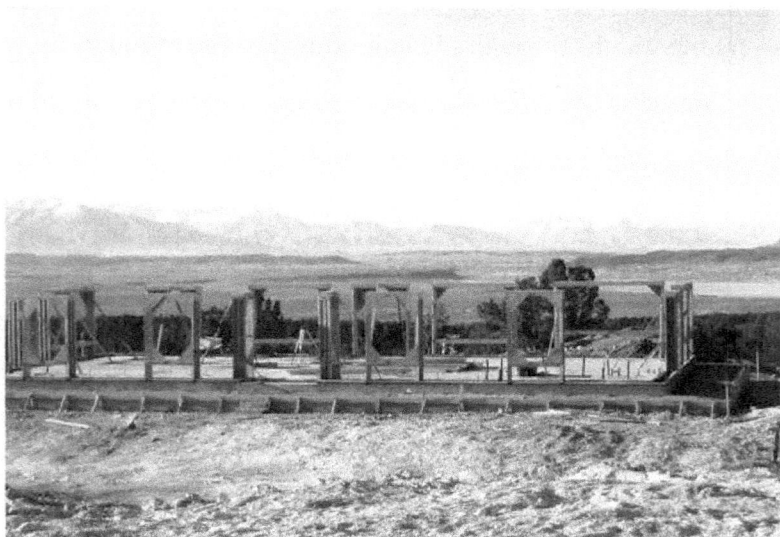

Window and door framing extends from the concrete foundation and span tops of doors and windows. Straw bales will be packed in between, beneath, and above the bucks. This style is called straw bale in-fill.

Some straw bale homes use bales under windows to support windows themselves. Given settling and weight considerations this may not be adequate, especially with larger windows. It is wise to frame windows from the foundation up and then put straw bales above window bucks as they will be solidly supported below by the concrete foundation. This leaves no chance for the weight of bales to mal-adjust or damage a window or its placement. Even better is to fake the look of bales above windows as some straw bale owners have done, by using chicken wire or lath tied to framing then stuffing the small space created between the lath and framing with straw. This avoids a weight load bearing on windows frames.

Packing bales tightly around posts, or 2" x 6" framing, is called straw bale in-fill. The bales fill-in between framing members or wall space and provide terrific insulation. This is the style I recommend for optimal structural integrity.

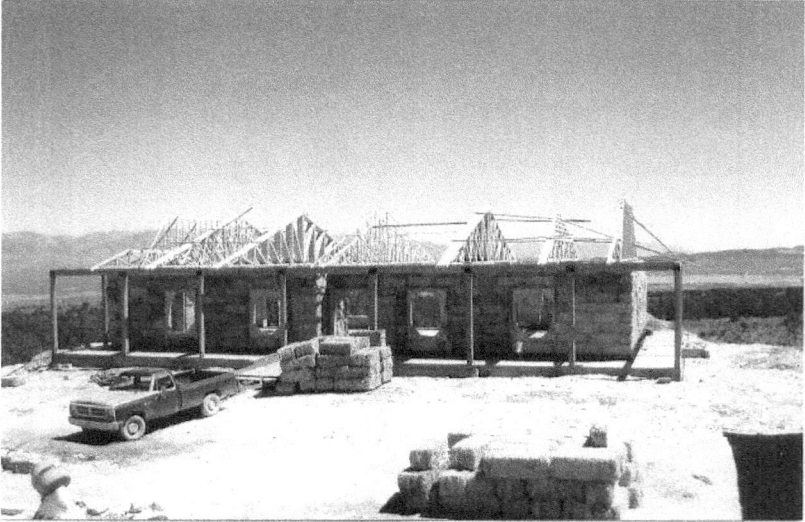

Straw bale in-filled walls; roof trusses rest on external post and beams, though trusses are not yet spread into place in this photo. Trusses will be attached to beams and top plates via Simpson seismic anchors. Notice the horizontal 2" x 4" bracing to hold trusses steady temporarily.

Foundations

There are four main types of foundations: monolithic slab; monolithic slab with stem walls; basement; and crawl space with stem walls.

The foundation style should depend upon home design, how much concrete or wood work you may or may not wish to do, and local building codes.

Monolithic slabs are favorable for the greatest amount of thermal mass heat retention. Thermal mass can also be had using tile over wood subfloors, but it will be less efficient. A monolithic slab is a foundation that is one solid piece – thus monolithic.

When pouring concrete for an average sized home solo or with a building partner it is next to impossible to pour everything - footings, thickened edges, and slab in just one day.

Concentrate on pouring solid footings first. Sometimes footings and stem walls must be poured together. Blue prints will specify this. If unsure, ask the building inspector or local concrete source how it's typically done in your area.

Once footings are poured and mostly cured pour concrete stem walls, or build stem walls from masonry blocks, mortar, rebar spaced vertically according to engineer specs, and fill with concrete. For the thickened edges and monolithic slabs pour no more than 1,000 square feet in one day – this is as much as two ordinary do-it-yourselfers can handle.

Crawl space foundations require footings and solid concrete stem walls, or concrete filled block stem walls. The top of the stem walls are framed up for walls and subflooring.

I will go into explicit detail on how to actually build foundation and all else in the next volume: *Creating a Green Home: Building a Straw Bale Cottage.*

Below are two common foundation types good for passive solar designs.

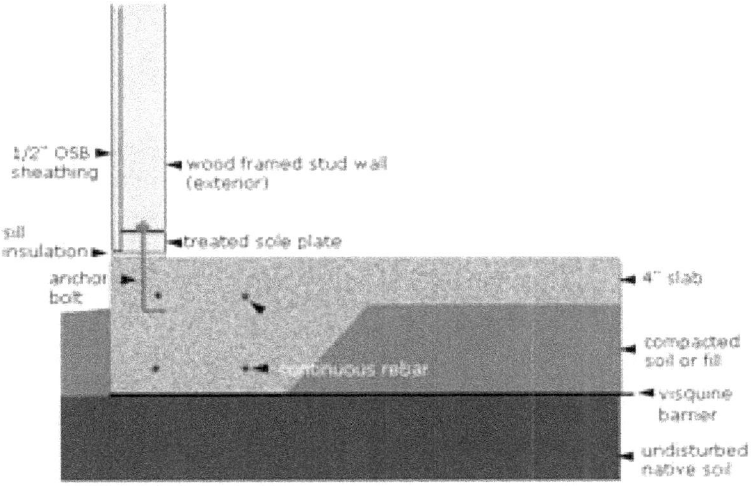
1/2" OSB sheathing
wood framed stud wall (exterior)
sill insulation
treated sole plate
anchor bolt
4" slab
compacted soil or fill
continuous rebar
visquine barrier
undisturbed native soil

Monolithic foundation cross-section

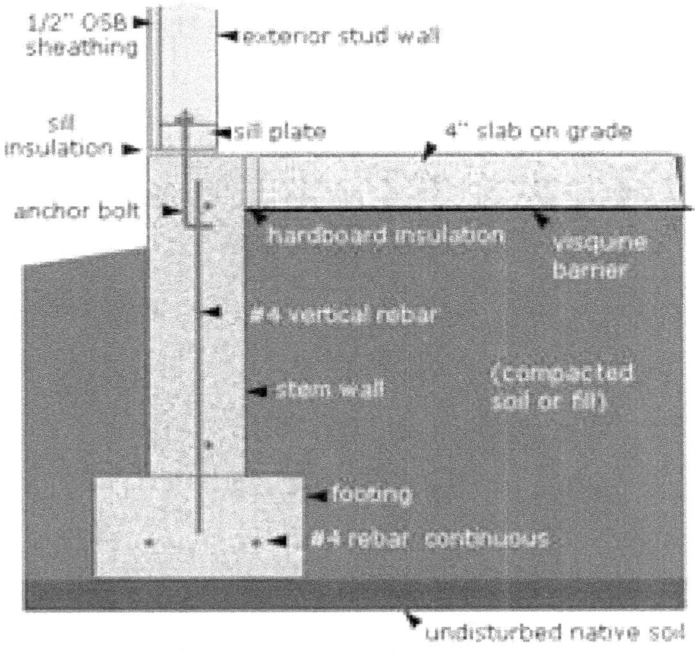
1/2" OSB sheathing
exterior stud wall
sill insulation
sill plate
4" slab on grade
anchor bolt
hardboard insulation
visquine barrier
#4 vertical rebar
stem wall
(compacted soil or fill)
footing
#4 rebar continuous
undisturbed native soil

Stem wall/slab foundation cross-section

Windows

Windows are important for light, heat, cooling, and mental health. Good windows are not cheap. Spend the money.

Passive solar design with a long south wall gracing the most used rooms connects inhabitants with the great outdoors. Use windows to seize expansive views and make time spent indoors more pleasant.

Big windows protect us from the elements while allowing us to view weather, wildlife, and the outdoor events. We can watch hawks, eagles, and blue birds fly above or perch; and autumn sunsets are sublime with their changing hues from green to orange to pink. Even if a view is of a cityscape or building capitalize on it. A home will feel more peaceful with views from as many rooms as possible.

Many who live in urban environments have lost touch with nature. It's time to reconnect – beginning with windows.

Buy super energy efficient well made windows. They save you money by reducing energy costs, feel better, and simply are more beautiful additions to a home than budget windows.

Vinyl windows, which are very popular now due to their low maintenance factor, are not environmentally sound. Vinyl off gasses toxins into interior and exterior environments. It is a phthalate, a known endocrine-disrupting chemical. Phthalates have been linked to breast cancer and early puberty in girls.

Look for Low-E glass, solid framing materials such as wood clad with metal, gas filled double or triple panes, and good weather stripping.

Solid metal framed windows are not good insulators against cold or heat. Metal transmits both hot and cold right into interior spaces.

When installing windows caulk and seal around edges well to prevent air infiltration. Caulking makes the building envelop tighter and more energy efficient in that it disallows drafts.

The following are some window glazing or glass performance, terms you should become familiar with when shopping for high quality windows.

U-Factor: U-factor measures how well a product prevents heat from escaping. The rate of heat loss is indicated in terms of the U-factor (U-value) of a window assembly. U-factor ratings generally fall between 0.20 and 1.20. The insulating value is indicated by the R-value, which is the inverse of the U-factor. The lower the U-factor, the greater a window's resistance to heat flow and the better its insulating value.

Solar Heat Gain Coefficient: Solar heat gain coefficient (SHGC) measures how well a product blocks heat caused by sunlight. The SHGC is the fraction of incident solar radiation admitted through a window, both directly transmitted and absorbed and subsequently released inward. SHCG is expressed as a number between 0 and 1. The lower a window's solar heat gain coefficient, the less solar heat it transmits.

Visible Transmittance: The visible transmittance (Vt) is an optical property that indicates the amount of visible light transmitted. Vt is expressed as a number between 0 and 1. The higher the Vt, the more light is transmitted.

Condensation Resistance Rating: Condensation Resistance (CR) measures how well a window or door resists the formation of condensation. CR is expressed as a number between 1 and 100. A higher number indicates better resistance to condensation.

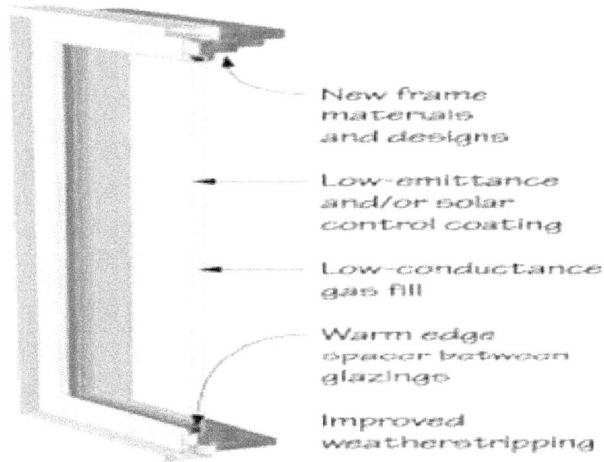

Labels from the diagram:
- New frame materials and designs
- Low-emittance and/or solar control coating
- Low-conductance gas fill
- Warm edge spacer between glazings
- Improved weatherstripping

The diagram above was taken from the Efficient Windows Collaborative website (www. efficient.windows.org) and shows construction elements of a quality window.

Decide upon window style or type. I recommend designing to account for no more than 2 window styles. Our home utilized casement windows and French doors. That's it.

Consistency in material types and styles lends one more harmonious element to a home. Building a home will be, after all, a grand opus. Compose each feature in accordance with its function and the overall home style in mind.

Casement windows have cranks or knobs that turn to open the windows along a vertical plain. This design captures and directs air flow better than other window styles.

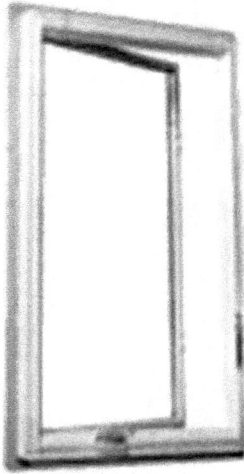

Casement window

Double-hung windows are also popular in that they slide up and/or down and often tilt open on a horizontal plain. New designs from some manufactures make at least one of the two pains easily removable for cleaning.

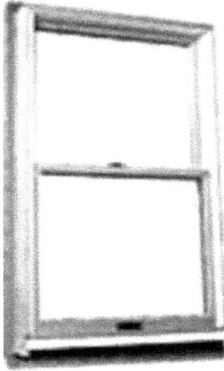

Double-hung window

Awning windows are similar to double-hung except there is only one pane and thus usually only one opening option.

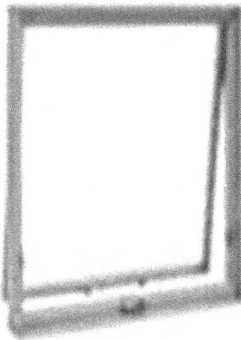

Awning window

Fixed windows that do not open are also called picture windows or plate glass windows. They can save money in areas where breezes emergency exits, or egress is not needed.

A good configuration to save money is to have one opening pane and one fixed pane which makes views larger, allows for breezes, but saves on the bottom line. Fixed windows are of course cheaper than windows that open.

Bedrooms must have egress windows in case of fire or other emergency so that people can actually fit through them. Check codes in your area or phone the local building inspector to see if egress windows are required anywhere else.

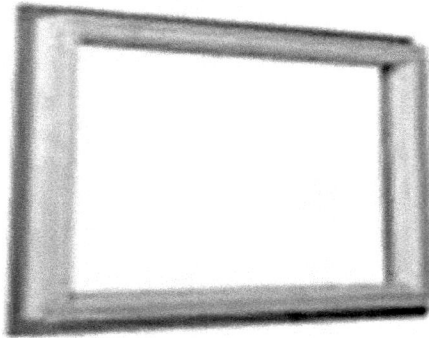

Picture window, fixed pane, or plate glass window

Sliding windows, often used in tract homes, should be a last choice. Window tracks quickly and easily become dirt filled which makes their operation less smooth. They also do not open out either vertically or horizontally to capture air flow guiding it into the home. Often sliders are the cheapest windows available from a manufacturer and there's a reason for it.

More windows allow more light to enter at different times of the day and change the way rooms look and feel. You are never limited to a view out one direction.

In our master bedroom with views to the south and east we can gaze at the eastern mountains as the sun rises and see how the mountains appear to change colors during fall's late day light, or look to the lake for a tranquil feel. Views of water are soothing.

Windows that look to the outside world allow a home's residents to connect with nature, whether the views are of expansive mountains, meadows, backyard gardens, or urban cityscapes.

Sill heights should be low enough so that when people are seated they can still see out. Sills heights approximately 2' above the finished floor height are usually good. Sill heights above 2' limit views. In snowy areas sill heights below 2' on the first floor of a home, will have snow piling up against windows during heavy storms or winter accumulations. Lower sill heights, below 1', may lend themselves to pets leaning against glass. If privacy from neighbors is a concern you may have to raise sill heights accordingly. Adjust your location, but generally lower will be better.

Roofs

Many straw bale homes have fairly simple roof lines since many are erected by owner-builders and accommodate simple, rectangular or square, home designs. Straw bale homes most often are right angled buildings, with few complexities, due largely to the rectangular prism shape of the bales.

Two main principles in straw bale design are: getting the bales up off of the grade of the land so that moisture of any sort cannot pool or remain against the lower portions of walls; and, getting the bales covered. I think of this as the Up and Covered principle of straw bale design. Here are some basic roof designs to consider that work nicely over straw bales or any other home:

A gable roof is the standard A-frame style roof. It works well on single and multi-story homes and is easy to put up. Trusses sit directly on framing between bales, post and beams, or the bales themselves in the case of load bearing walls. A gable roof lends itself easily to having covered porches or nice overhangs on at least two sides of the house, and many designs incorporate lower "shed" roofs on the gabled ends if they want more entries or straw bale walls covered well.

Similar to the gable and shed idea is a box gable where the gabled ends are extended out away from the house with siding as fascia and a soffit beneath.

Dutch gable roofs are attractive and offer coverage well on all four sides of a building.

Any roof can serve to cover a wrap-around porch as long as its weight or "load" is supported adequately.

Another nice style roof, but one that may not work as well for passive solar overhangs, is a simple shed roof. A shed roof is one sided slope, and has a wonderful modern, rustic, or classic appearance depending upon your application and home style.

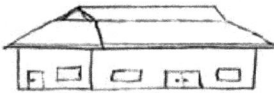

Dutch Gable Roof

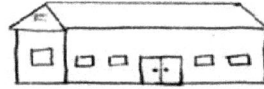

Common Gable Roof

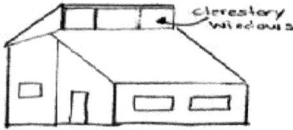

Double Shed Roof

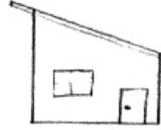

Shed Roof

Clerestory Windows

Different roof styles and looks. You can combine more than one style into your home, but be prepared for more complex construction and time to build

Most reading this likely live in areas where flat roofs will not work well due to snow loads or rains. Flat roofs fit well with the southwestern style of many straw bale homes, but a slight slope and drainage must be incorporated into the design.

Roof pitches are generally referred to by a ratio called rise to run. Our roof is a "4 on 12" or 4:12 pitch; which means that the roof rises 4" over a horizontal linear distance of 12" and equally rises 4' over a horizontal distance of 12'.

Roofs of 0:12 - 2:12 are considered flat roofs. Low roofs have 2:12 – 4:12 rises. Most conventional roofs have 4:12 – 9:12 rises; and higher than 9:12 are steep roofs.

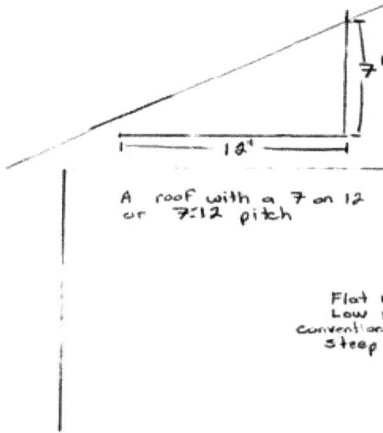

A roof with a 7 on 12
or 7:12 pitch

Flat roof   0:12 – 2:12
Low roof   2:12 – 4:12
Conventional roof 4:12 - 9:12
Steep roof   9:12 and higher

**Above is a diagram showing 7:12, this can be viewed as either rising 7"
for every 12" or 7' for every 12**

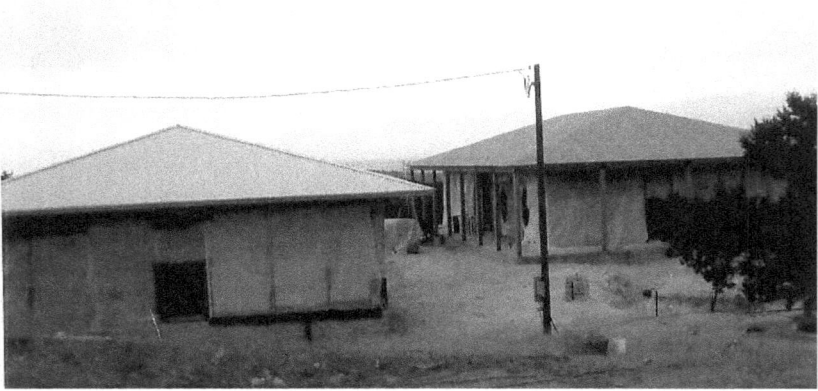

A pyramid roof over the straw bale garage and hip roof on the main house

There are numerous roofing materials available: asphalt/ composite shingles, standing seam and corrugated metals, tile, slate, cedar... Slate and cedar roofs may be more expensive and not necessarily green or in keeping with energy efficient designs.

Spanish-Ranch style homes with tile roofs do not necessarily do well in areas with high winds, can be expensive, and do not reflect heat. Choose roof materials wisely and in keeping with overall architectural style.

Consider a rain water capture system from the roof. We didn't install rain barrels or the like since our roof edges drip onto planted or landscaped areas, but not all gardens are immediately surrounding the home. If water is captured and stored, it can be dispersed to garden areas elsewhere.

Rain water capture may be simple, like with rain barrels, or far more complex and time consuming to install with capture tanks (barrels or other tanks), filtration, and exterior plumbing to garden or water use areas.

Ceiling Heights

Consider the functions of interior spaces and their corresponding ceilings heights. Varying ceiling heights may better suit individual room purposes and appeal to you. Often people choose to put higher ceilings in living rooms or large common areas, and lower ceilings over dining areas, kitchens, or bathrooms.

Many designers would suggest lower ceilings over such areas as dining rooms or breakfast nooks to create feelings of greater intimacy. This is fine if conversation after dinner is mostly enjoyed more quietly, or amongst only a few people. Yet, more often than not dinner party conversations tend to migrate into living rooms or common rooms that offer greater comfort, space, and views. Dining spaces that have higher ceilings invite people to stay longer because they simply feel more comfortable.

Rooms with heightened ceilings have more air to breathe, feel expansive, and more relaxed than the same square footage with standard 8' ceilings. We have found that in a home with 12' ceilings throughout, people feel good remaining in any given room or space for extended periods of time. There's never a feeling of having to leave the table, or other location, to move to a more comfortable area.

Higher ceilings cost more money due to more linear board feet of lumber. A 1,400 square foot home with 8' ceilings costs less than the same house with 10' ceilings, which of course adds 2 ft. to every vertical framing member. Taller rooms use more straw bales and likely have longer wiring and plumbing runs – which means more wiring and pipes. Compare costs, but usually adding a foot, or two, or four, here or there to achieve a grander feel, have more air to breath, and make rooms feel better is worth the extra cost.

Too small rooms with low ceilings, or small rooms with ceilings that are disproportionately high, feel awkward. It is important to visualize and imagine spaces. As you consider ceiling heights begin closely examining and *feeling* the spaces you currently occupy. Closely analyze spaces in your current home, friends' houses or apartments, commercial buildings, everywhere you go. I recommend reading home design books and magazines such as Architectural Digest and others. Which ceiling heights look and feel great to you? Design and build what will function best and feel fabulous.

If building a straw bale home, keep in mind that higher ceilings require higher straw bale walls. You will likely hand lug, carry, drag, and haul bales to the top of the walls. This requires scaffolding or a stacking of other bales upon which to climb. Bales are not light and often placement requires two people.

Baled wall height will not be perfect to the inch as per your blue prints so you will have to split open bales and use flakes for getting that extra few inches. You will want to go a little higher than your planned finished height since bales will be tightly compressed later on.

Main Entry

Whether a home is small, large, or somewhere in between an entry that separates you or visitors from the weather, the street, and world outside your home - be it a busy sidewalk or unpopulated hillside – is highly desirable. An exterior entry must allow for a porch or roof covering to keep precipitation off people at the door, and provide place to feel sheltered and separated from the open environment. A sheltered entry provides the first break from the outside world before entering interior space.

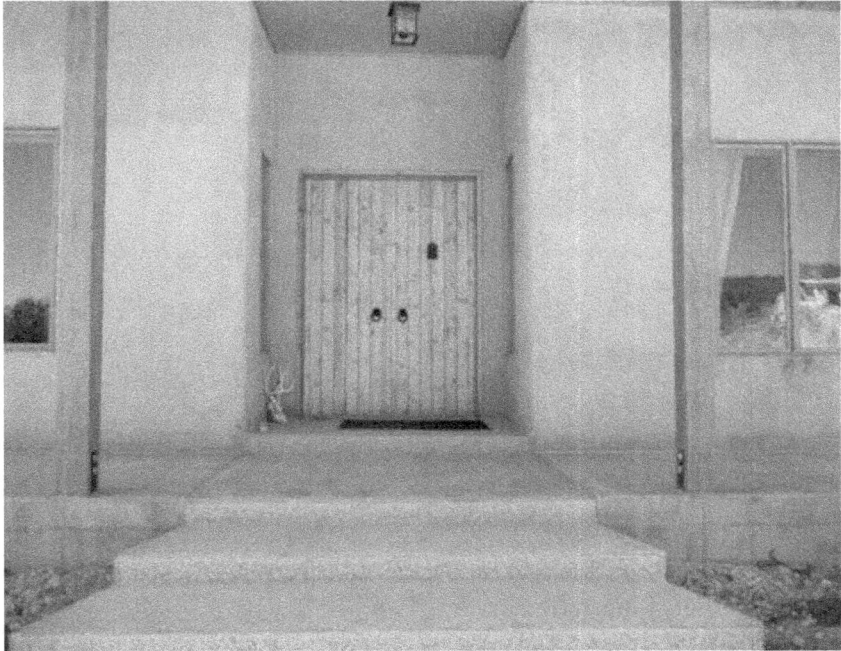

The exterior front entry allows visitors to separate physically and psychologically from the outside world

The second break from the outside is an entry room that allows for taking off boots, hanging coats in a closet, and setting down bundles once the entry door is closed. This space should not be part of a main common room, like the living room or kitchen, in that delivery people or others who may just step a foot inside need not be privy to the more private residence.

Remember that form follows function and the entry should be its own space for its designed purpose – to put on or take off coats and shoes, greet visitors, and to physically and psychologically prepare us for entry or exit to or from the outside.

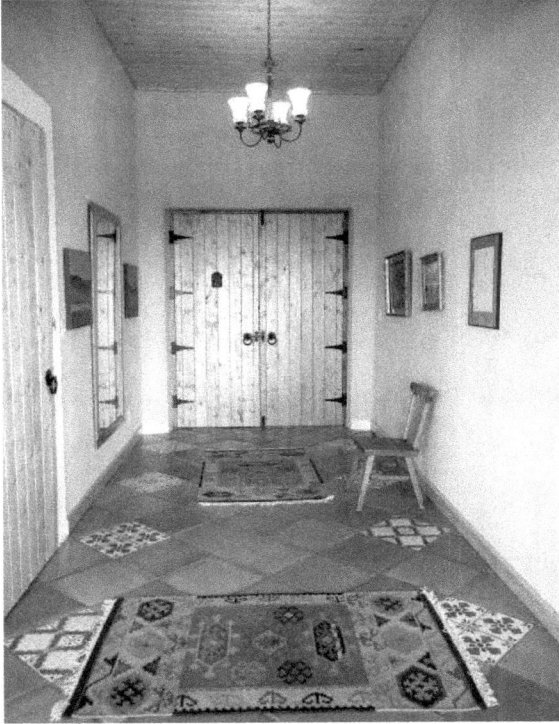

The front entry space doubles as an art gallery. The large vertical mirror on the left wall offers a place for a final appearance check before entering or leaving. Rob made all the pine doors out of tongue and groove pine.

Kitchens and Common Areas

There's a saying that the kitchen is the heart of the home. Design your kitchen to match your personal cooking style. Chefs need work surfaces, tools readily at hand, and good ventilation. In the kitchen, this means plenty of counter space, well thought out storage, room to move, and operable windows on at least two sides.

Kitchen counter height should allow the chef to easily use upper body weight or strength for downward pressure when chopping food, but not be so low that he/she has to hunch or bend. To determine how high a counter top should be bend your arms at the elbows a little greater than 90 degrees, so that forearms slope down very slightly. Imagine you are using a knife or rolling out dough. Measure from the floor to the palms of your hands and this height will be a great counter top height for you. My kitchen counter tops are 38 1/4" h from finished floor, higher than the standard 36"h.

Raising standard cabinets and the consequent counter heights is achieved simply by constructing toe-ups, 2" x 4" or 2" x 6" lumber laid flat under cabinet edges and nailed to subflooring. I'll provide more information on construction details in Part II of *Creating a Green Home: Building a Straw Bale Cottage*

One kitchen design option is a kitchen with work zones, or areas that accommodate a specific purpose. This way a chef can organize tools and materials in each area for easy access and functionality. I designed my kitchen with zones and it has proven a highly functional and practical design. The work areas are ergonomic, spacious, and pleasant.

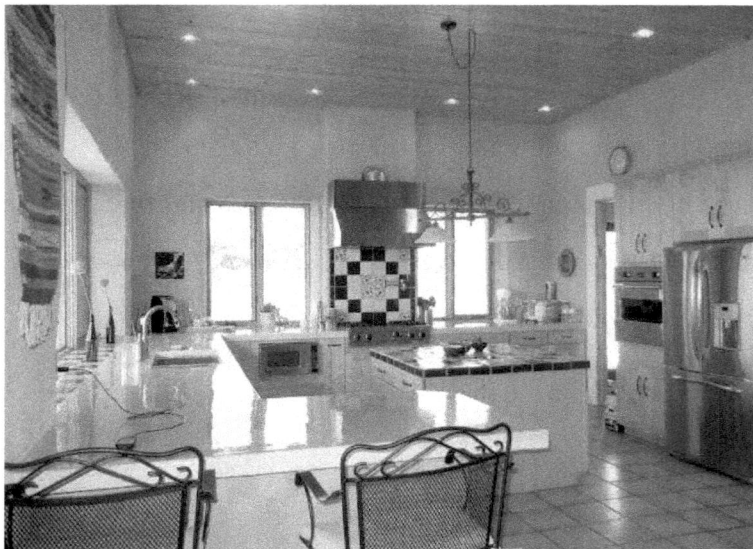

This kitchen was designed with work zones in mind.

The old philosophy of reducing steps in the kitchen strikes me as a physically unhealthy way to cook. Standing in one place makes one tired, the work tedious, and it's physically unhealthy. Chefs were meant to move!

Decide upon cabinet type and placement carefully. Hanging or wall cabinets give a kitchen a heavier, lower-ceiling feel than a kitchen without wall cabinets. Kitchen space feels more open and airy with only base cabinets. But, if you have trouble bending or squatting to reach into low base cabinets, wall cabinets would be better for your individual needs.

I designed a kitchen where the cook can enjoy views out two directions, with no hanging cabinets on exterior walls. All base cabinets have roll-out shelves for easy access. The kitchen feels much larger than it is and makes cooking or just hanging out enjoyable.

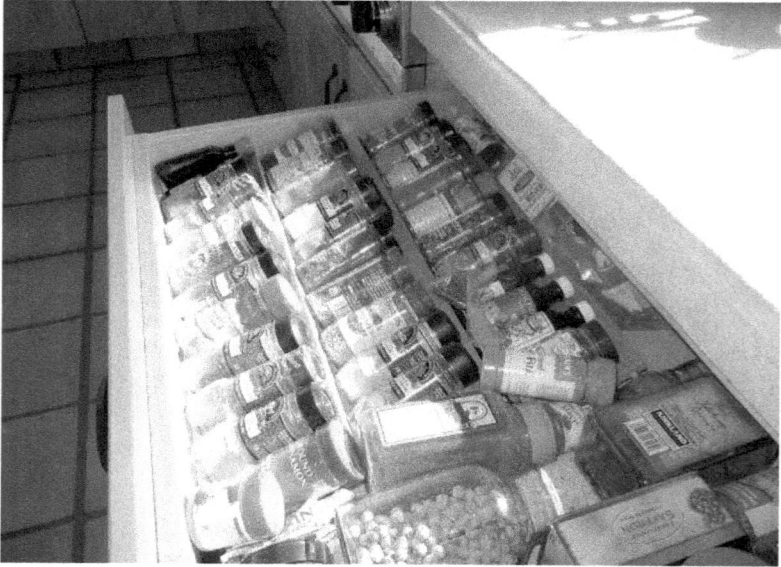

This spice drawer insert is to the immediate right of the range top
to serve stove top and baking area needs.

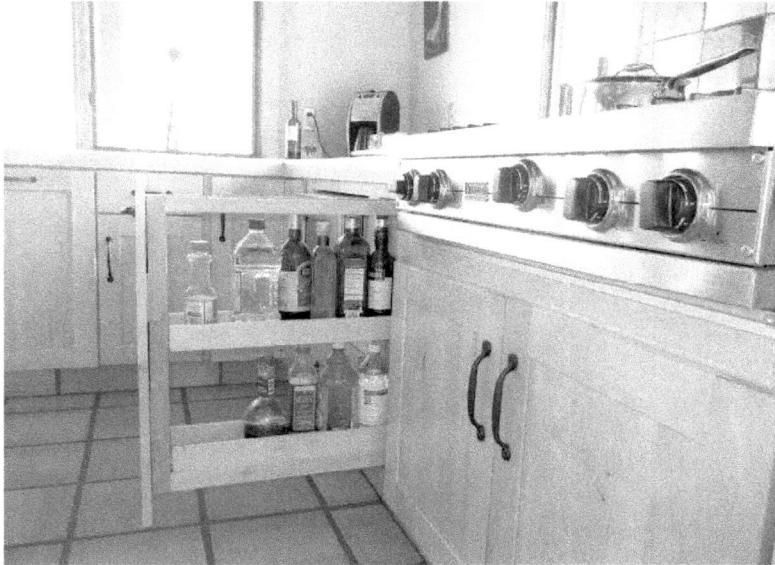

**A pullout bottle bin next to the range helps
organize oils and cooking wines**

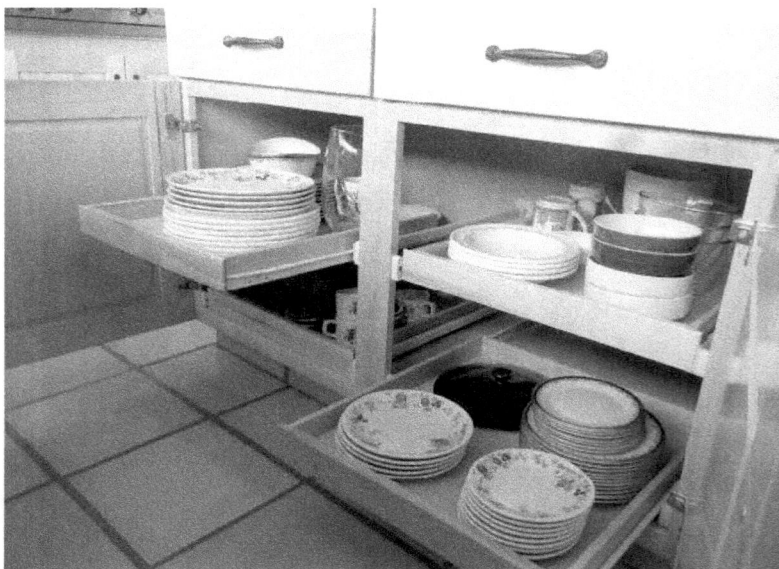

Roll out shelves in the island hold dishes

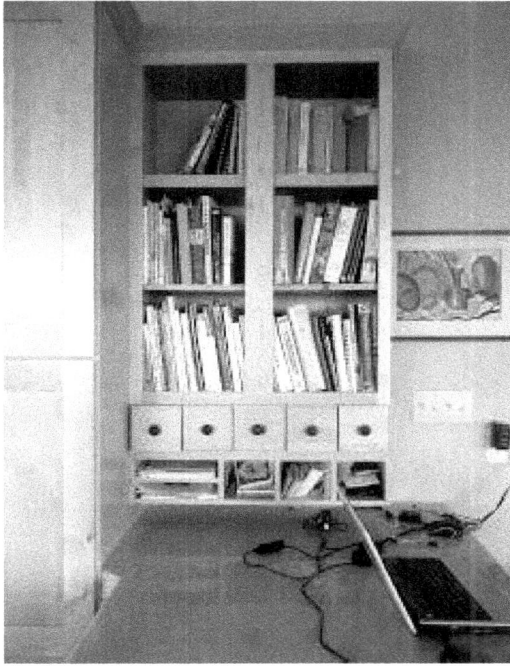

Cookbook shelves at a work station in the kitchen area

We chose to install counter tops without any seems or grout lines. For us this meant concrete, but solid granite, marble, hard woods, or other sheet type surfaces would work too. Concrete counter tops require sealing with either a wax or epoxy.

Bees' wax is a natural, safe, semi-gloss sealant, but is susceptible to stains from such things as coffee and red wine. Plus bees' wax is permeable and holds bacteria making it less sanitary than sealing with epoxy. The downside of epoxy sealant is that it is toxic while wet, however once dry it is perfectly safe and seals a counter top well – impervious to staining or bacterial penetration – thus it's more sanitary than bees' wax.

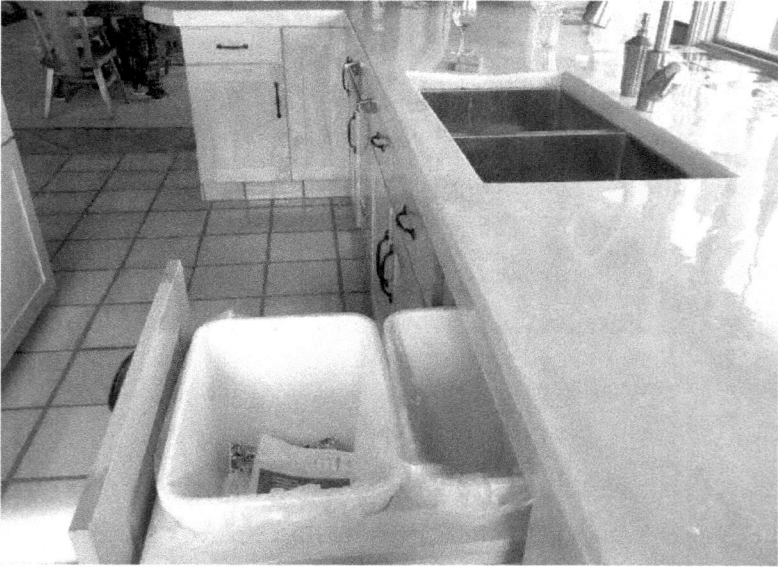

Seamless counter tops: To the right of the sink, just beneath the vegetable chopping area is a trash and compost bin pull out.

Concrete counter tops, pictured here, were made using white cement and left over American Clay color pigment. The counter tops are really only about 2" deep on top, but we built a drop down on the front edge of the concrete forms to give a thicker appearance of about 3". Base cabinet sides were built stouter using stronger plywood to support concrete weight. Notice the built-in drain board to the left of the sink so no dish rack is needed. Concrete is fun to work with.

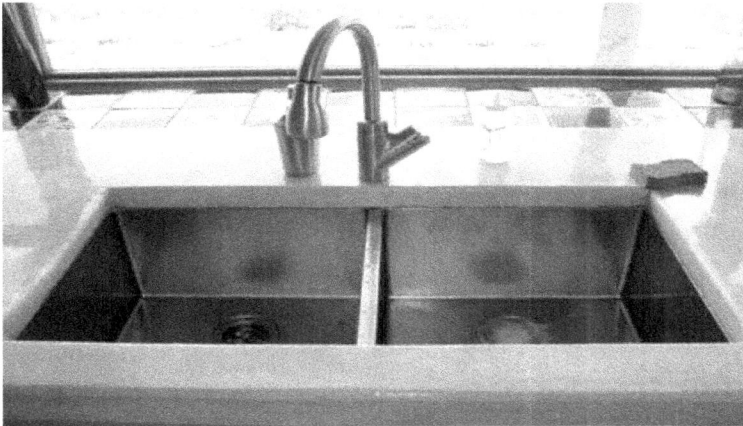

A nice deep, 12 in. sink with built in drain board to left, made by shaping concrete to slope into sink

Family and guests like to gather near where food is being prepared or beverages are easily had. Allow gathering space in or adjacent to kitchen space to allows socializing with the chef(s). Perhaps have a counter area for hors d'oeurves or nashes.

Make sure the common area of the home is centrally located, or at the heart. This space should have southern exposure for plenty of natural light, an open area for people to gather or mill about, as well as nooks or small seating areas where people may hold quiet conversations.

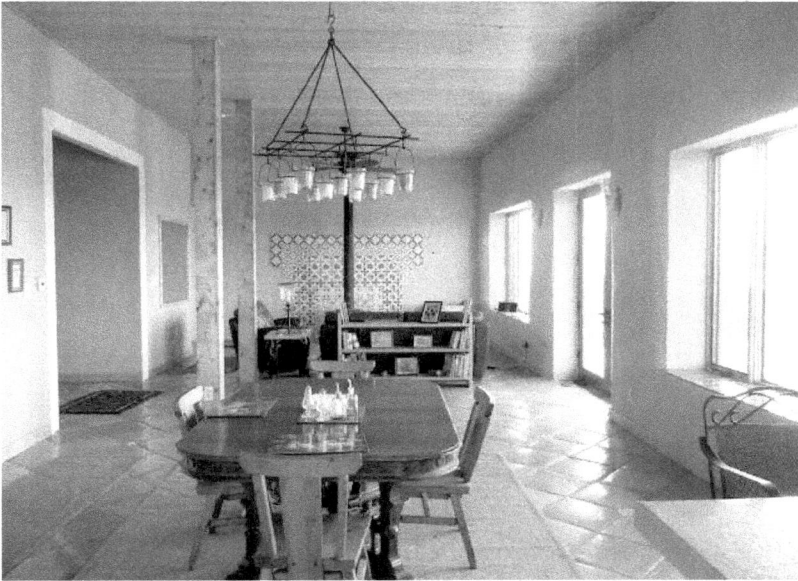

Photo taken from kitchen looking out to soul of home: South facing windows allow plenty of natural light; the chef can commune with guests seated at the table; vertical posts help divide room spaces.

Notice in the previous photo there are two columns utilized as psychological and physical barriers between the main entry and larger living area. The columns add a vertical visual element to break up a long and relatively narrow room, 55'l x 16'w. These columns also serve a utilitarian purpose: both hide and house wiring to outlets on the posts. Electrical outlets on each allow for plugging in a living room lamp, vacuum, computer, or whatever while sitting in the dining or living room areas.

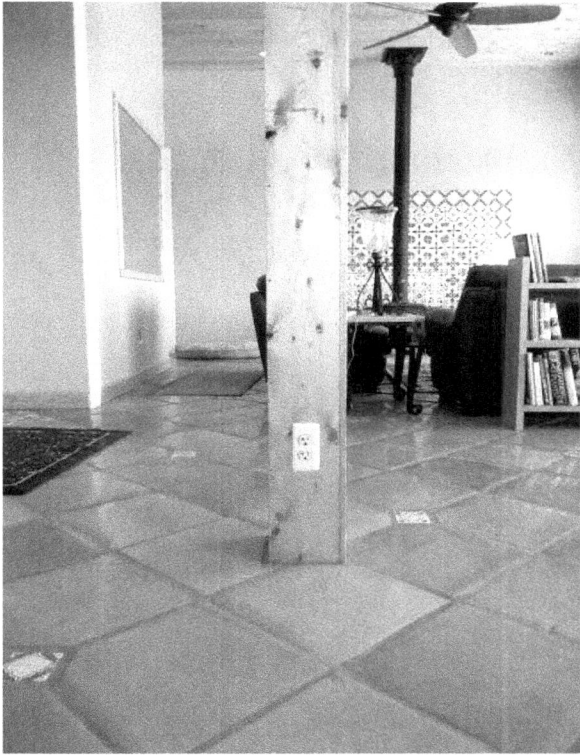

This decorative post serves to break up a large open space and as an electrical chase to run wiring from ceiling to outlet

Straw bale walls lend themselves as ideal window seats. Window sills can be tiled, plastered, covered with wood moldings or other decorative and durable finish materials.

Tiled or other dense materials on window seats can contribute to thermal mass and offer nice warm places to sit or gather with friends. We used terra cotta colored tile to absorb the sun's heat and radiate it back into rooms. The sills offer nice warm seats during winter months despite all the seemingly cold glass.

Sill areas and seats also serve as conversation nooks. Guests can pair or group to chat with a view of the goings on in the open room or to the outdoors. Adjacent to these nooks or larger open spaces should be columns, half walls, doorways or other subtle marks of leaving one space and entering another.

Passageways for entering a home and between rooms ought to have thickened edges noticeably marking or delineating exits and entries from one area to another. Thickened thresholds add greater impressions of permanence to a structure. Envision 2"w x ½"d door moldings as opposed to 10"w x 2"d. Of course the latter takes more material and costs a bit more, but offers much richer aesthetics.

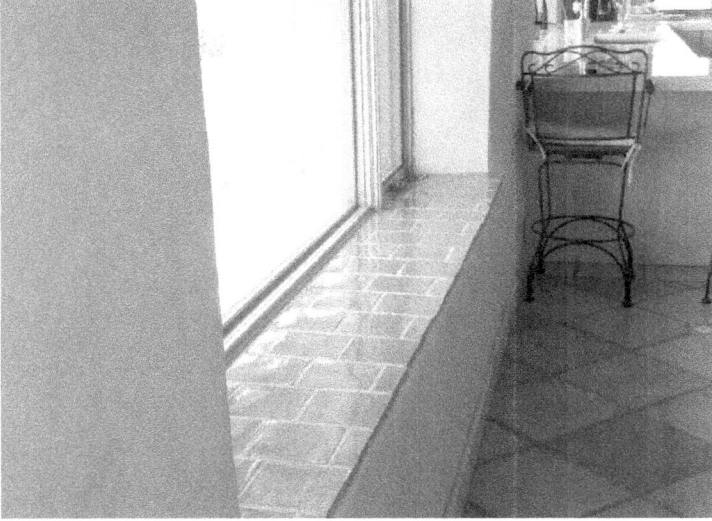
A natural window seat within the dining room

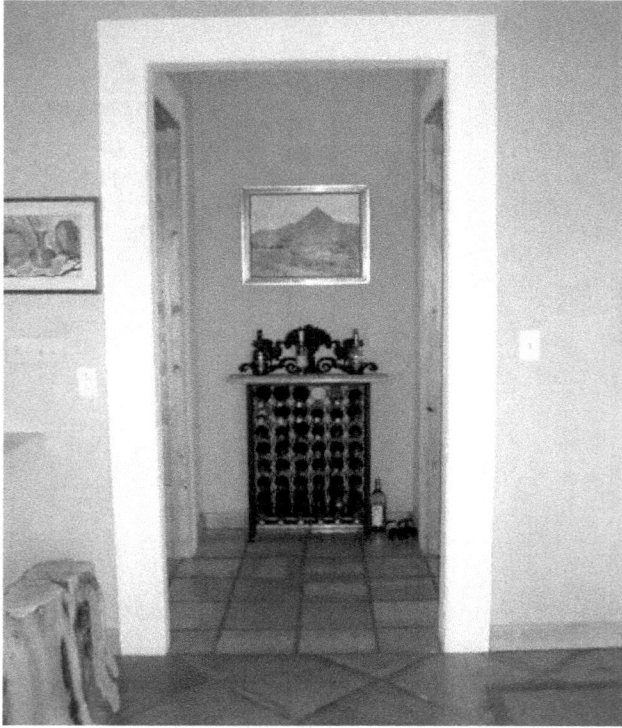

This passage way leads to a guest bedroom on right and bathroom on left, has thickened edges made with sheetrock and clay paint to frame the opening almost like a painting itself

Bedroom Privacy

Most people enter master suites or bedroom areas during regular daytime hours only to use the bathroom, take a sweater from a closet, or change clothes. These activities do not require actually being in the bedroom, but rather the bathroom, dressing room, or closet areas. The bedroom itself becomes a much nicer sanctuary when it is not a thoroughfare and when it's designed with its primary purposes in mind.

Given this, consider having the master suite entry area flow into a dressing area adjacent to the bedroom. The dressing area may be within a larger bathroom, which I show here in the following photos, or through a double sided closet pathway, or other floor plan layout.

Make a bedroom look and feel like a private enclave. If the bathroom and/or dressing area is separate, even guests can use these areas without breeching truly private space.

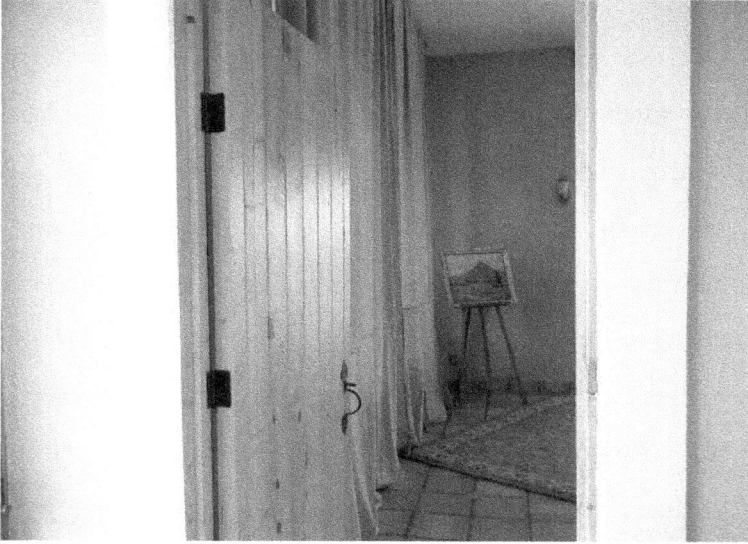

**A passage from master bath and dressing area into the bedroom;
There's no need for guests to ever enter such private space.**

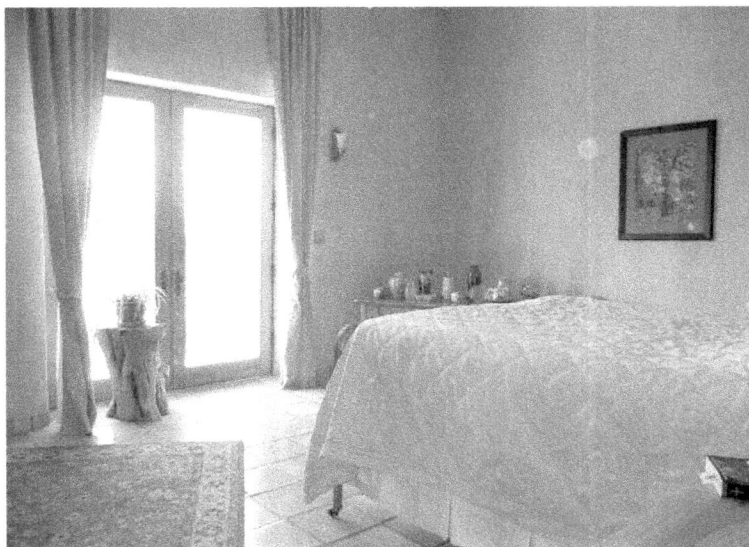

A master bedroom with a view

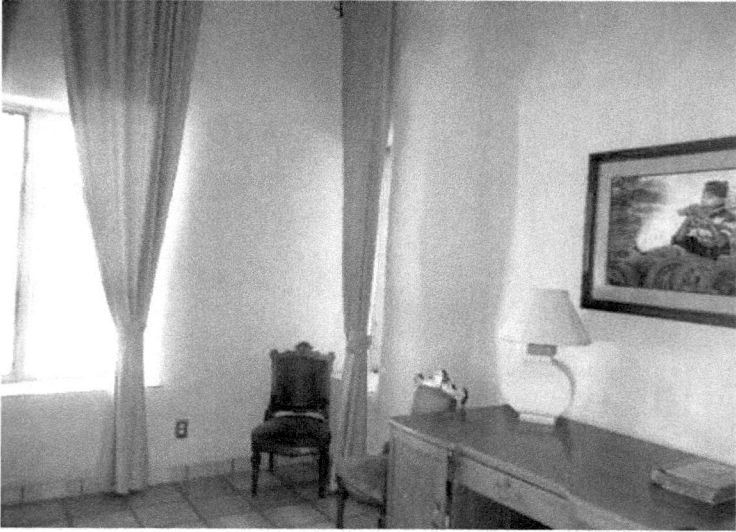

Guest accommodations allow visitors to use a desk in privacy

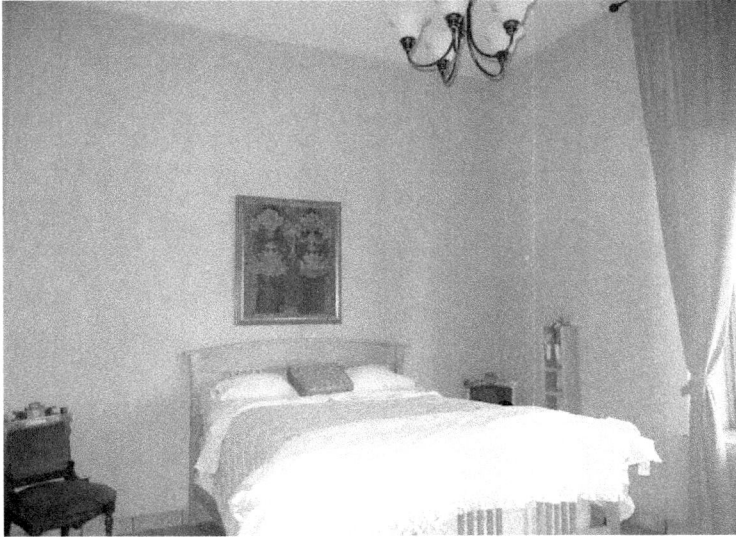

Thick straw bale exterior walls offer guests a more insulated and warm feeling

Bathrooms

Bathrooms are utilitarian rooms for bathing, showering, grooming, and dressing. These rooms, to be optimally functional, must afford room to move about. Make bathrooms rooms, rather than large closets with plumbing. Decide how often and for what purpose you'll be using specific bathrooms and design accordingly. Bathrooms serve important functions and should have the floor space and ergonomic layout to accommodate more than one user performing different tasks at a time.

Showering and bathing feels good. Most of us enjoy feeling clean, warming tired muscles, or simply having a large enough space to wash our hair and shave. Bathing is physically active and demands space! Make showers and tubs roomy. Large double walk-in showers and baths don't have to cost a fortune.

Walk-in showers can be simply small framed mini-rooms sheathed with cement board, rather than dry wall, then tiled. Notice in the next photos that a stock tank, or horse trough, was used as a bathtub. A Kohler or other good quality cast iron and enameled tubs cost hundreds and sometimes thousands of dollars. The stock tank cost a little more than $100. If opting for stock tanks, make sure you use thinset mortar beneath to slope the floor under the tub to the drain area otherwise water will pool slightly.

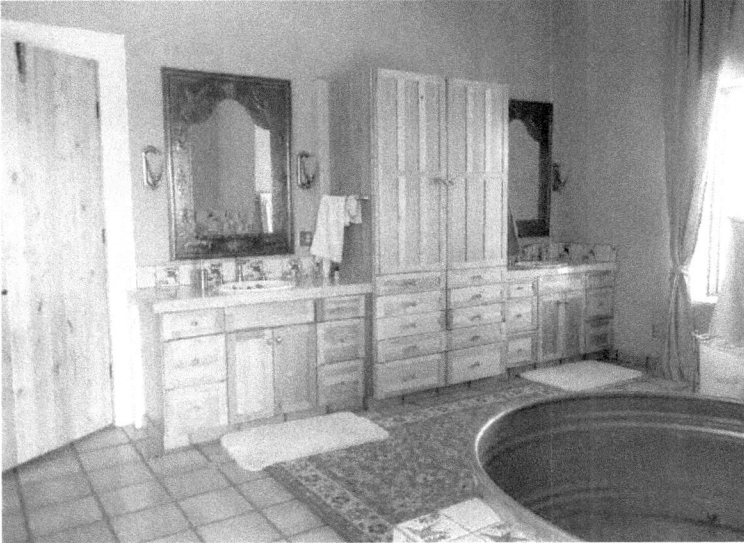

His and her basins and cabinets that afford linen storage,
clothing drawers, and room to dress

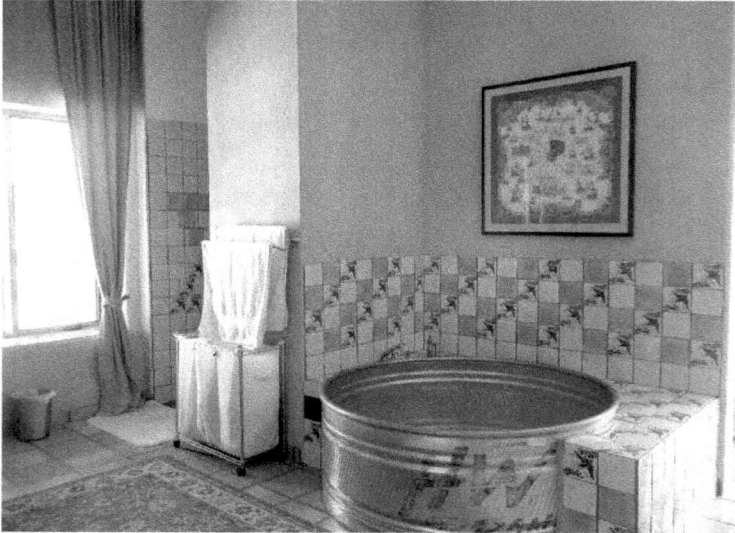

HW stock tank as bath tub; Kohler or other good quality bathtubs can cost $1,800 and up. Stock tank: $120.

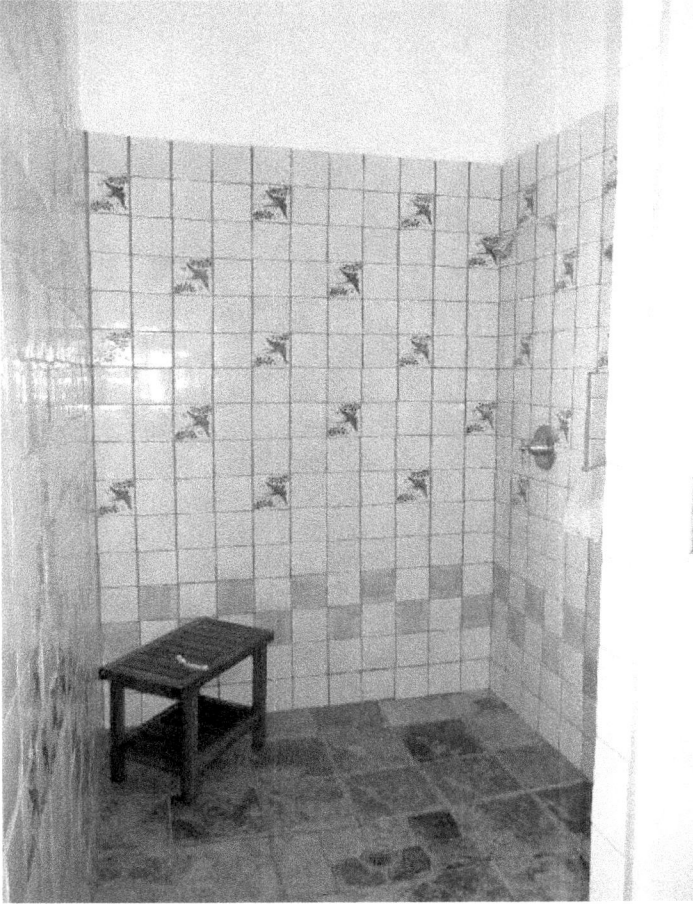

A master shower large enough for two to shower simultaneously under two separate shower heads, with entry wide enough for possible wheel chair access and an ADA approved grab bar (not shown).

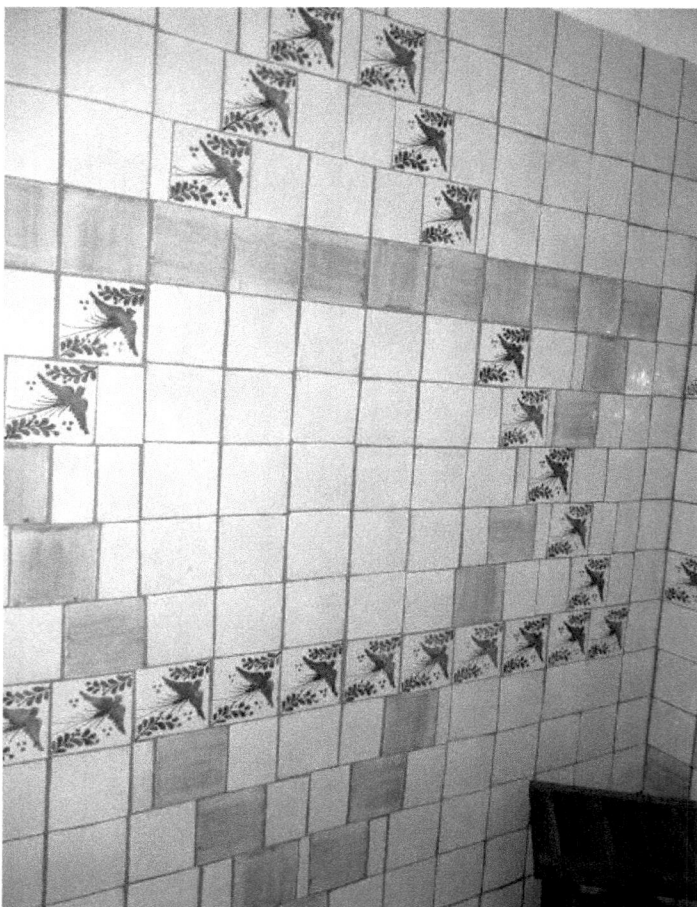

The Star of David tile layout, in birds and solids, reflects Rob's family heritage. Tile design should be done on graph paper to scale, before laying out on walls or floor.

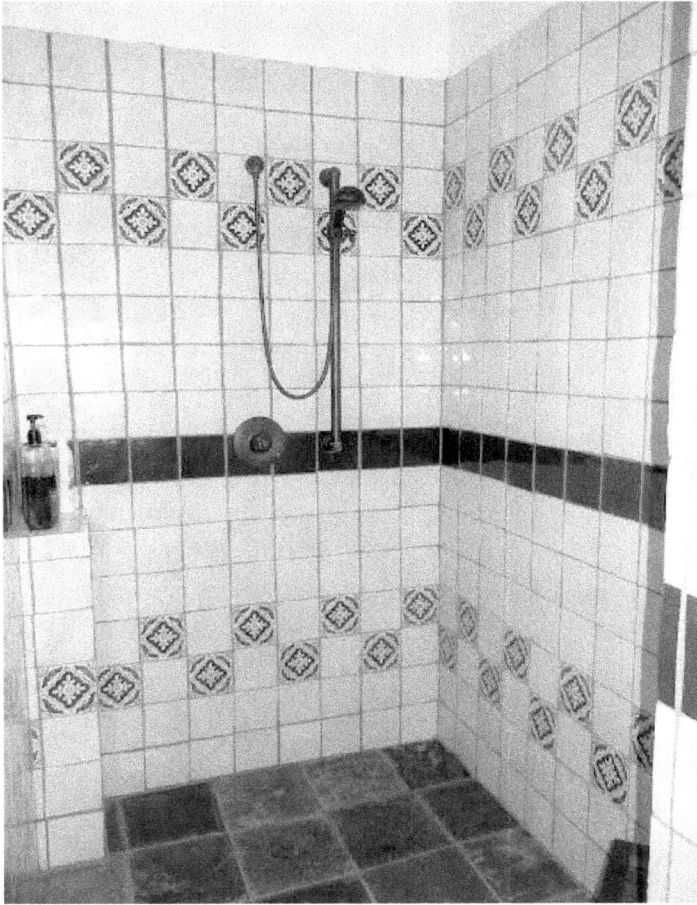

Slate tile floor and Talavera walls make this 5' x 6' shower

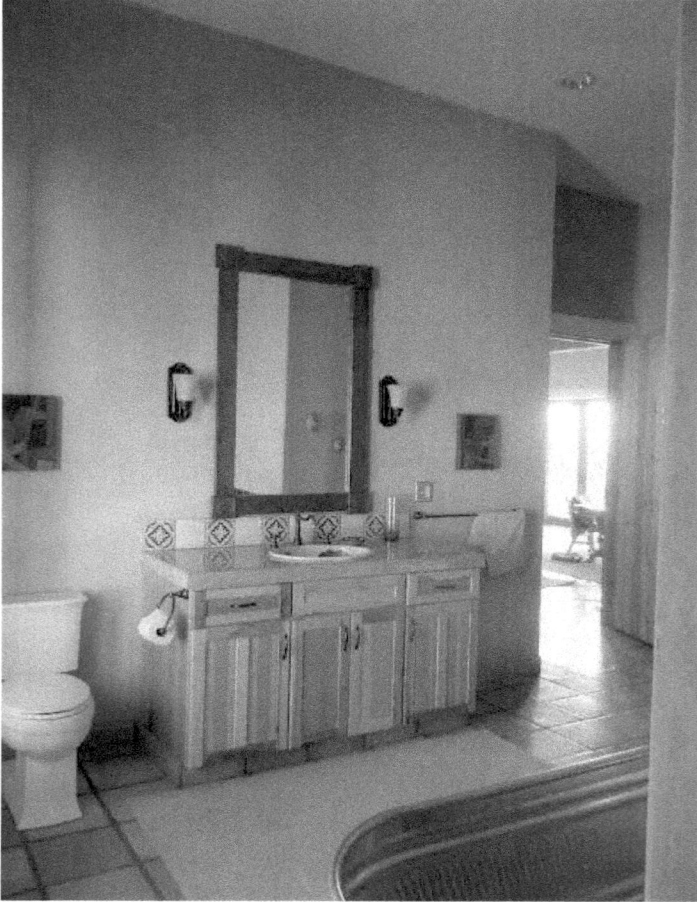

The open door in this bathroom illustrates breeze pathways throughout the house. Notice another stock tank as bathtub in foreground.

Storage

Most of us have far more stuff than we need. I suggest donating or just tossing most of it. Nevertheless, there are belongings that we cherish and others that we must have to run our daily lives, and they need a place within the home. Having adequate storage spaces, especially in utilitarian rooms like kitchens, baths, and laundry requires closets or cabinetry.

Linen and towel storage is necessary in or near bathrooms and bedrooms. You may want a large closet in the bathroom for dressing right from the shower, or a separate room for clothing.

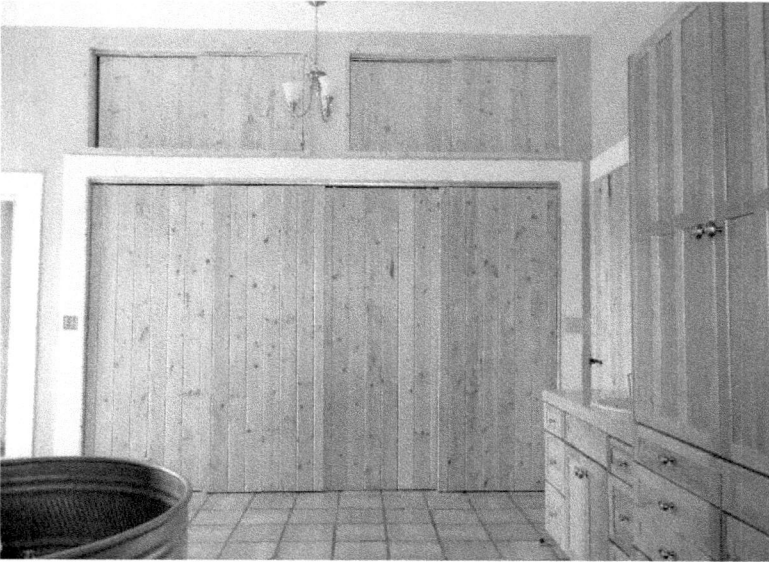

A 13 ft. long closet in the master dressing and bath area has built in racks and dowels to make the most of closet space. Avoid walk-in style closets as they make for wasted and dark space.

Closet organizer kits are easily purchased at the local hardware store. Closet organizers provide hanging, shelf, and drawers if needed maximizing closet space.

I usually advise against walk-in closets as most of them prove the epitome of poor design. They rarely have adequate lighting to see everything clearly, don't have room to physically move around to either dress or look for items, and most never have windows to allow in light or fresh air so they absorb shoe odors, mustiness, and more.

The preceding closet photo is of a 13'l by 30"d closet space. It has closet organizers that include top and bottom dowels for hanging clothes, and pull out drawers fro sweaters and such. The sliding storage doors above the main closet house little used luggage, extra blankets, and other occasional use items.

Kitchens need plenty of cupboard space for foods and cooking utensils. A laundry room needs a place for detergents and other household supplies like light bulbs, other cleaning supplies, and household tools. Main entry areas need coat closets where shoes and boots can be stored out of the way.

A kitchen panty room-closet is always great for additional dry good storage or maybe even indoor freezer space.

Windows on Two Sides of Every Room

Rooms feel better when we have a view and/or air circulation from two different directions. Rooms that accommodate windows on at least two walls are brighter, requiring less artificial lighting, offer breeze pathways, and make inhabitants feel better. There is a psychological affect with having views and air flow options.

We have windows on two sides of all rooms except two, the laundry room which has a glass door to the outside, and the guest bathroom which has 4'9" x 6' primary window so allows plenty of natural light. When guests comment about how good this home feels, one of the reasons is all the windows. Connecting with the natural world as much as possible, even through a window, makes us feel better.

Hallways

I advise against hallways as they take up usable room space. Challenge yourself to design a home without hallways. Hallways almost always account for wasted space.

Look at the next floor plan graphic. The laundry room, guest bathroom, bedroom, library, and master suite areas simply flow out of the common room spaces without hallways. There are no pathways to interrupt conversational areas in the middle of rooms. All pathways from room to room flow at edges or corners so as not to traverse or interrupt gathering spots.

Smaller room spaces should flow off of larger common areas for a series of continually smaller or more intimate spaces.

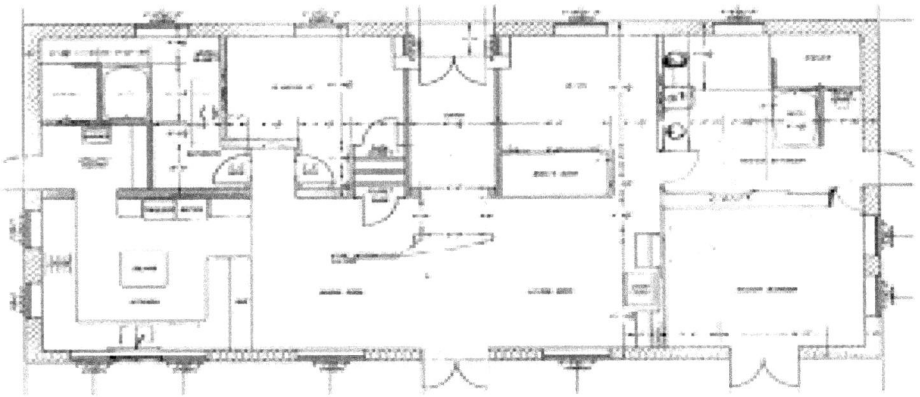

A home without hallways

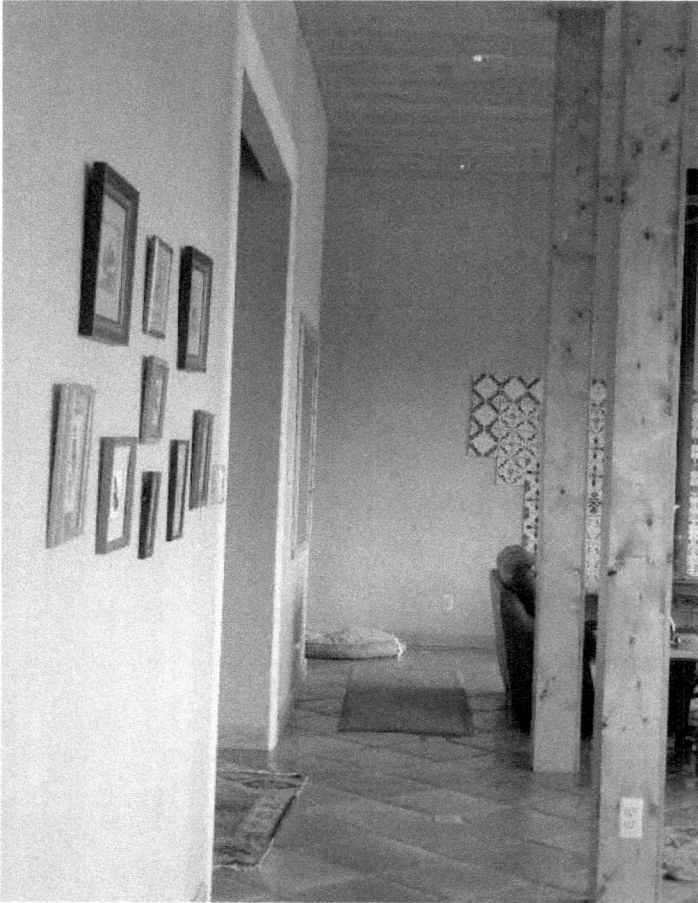

This corridor is a relative of a hallway. It does not block light or air flow, feel narrow, waste space.

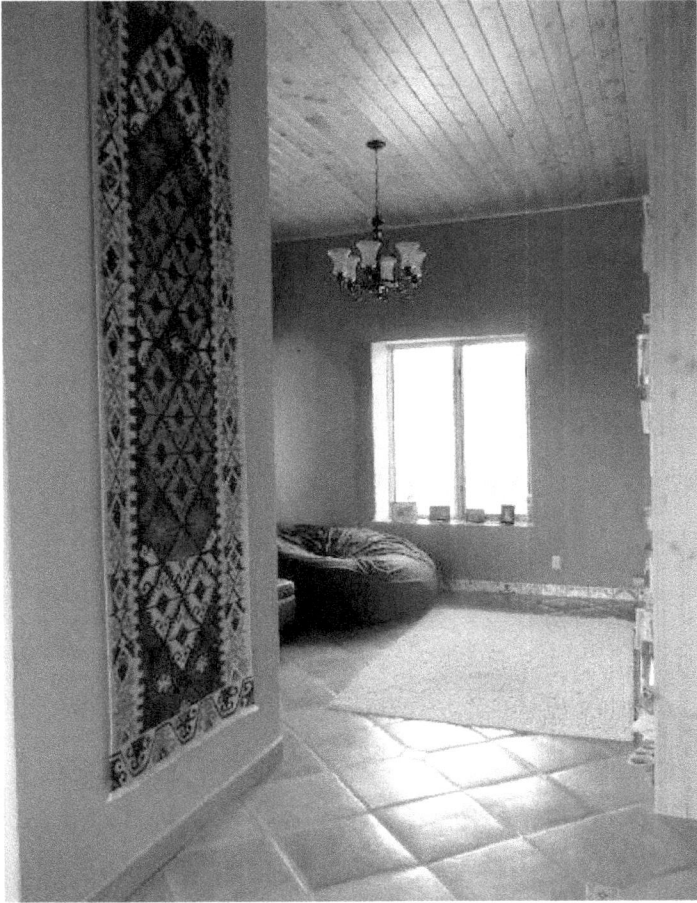

This smaller room off of the main living area affords a spot for people to talk quietly, or flop and read a book.

Indoor Air Quality

Install exhaust fans that are vented to the outside. Avoid fans that filter air back into the interior space. Some will argue that fans vented to the outside also vent hard earned or gained heat out during winter months. Forget about it. Non-toxic air is more important. Exhaust fans keep indoor air quality healthier by eliminating microbe carrying mold spores, smoke from cooking, bathroom moisture, and any possible toxic off-gassing to the outside.

Good quality fans are well worth the extra money. They run more smoothly, more powerfully, and are significantly quieter. Loud bathroom or kitchen fans rarely get used and indoor air must be vented to the outside regularly for optimal air quality. Most contemporary homes have so many toxic elements that, more often than not, indoor air quality is worse than outdoor pollution.

I cringed when I learned the price of my kitchen exhaust hood. I thought twice about buying it. Now after five years, I realize it was worth every penny. It's powerful, the motor mounted on the exterior of the wall makes it quieter, and it sucks so powerfully even on the low setting that we have to turn it off if we want to start a fire in the wood stove because the stove won't draft properly. The house air is fresh. With super energy efficient homes, heating is more or less free anyway, so rid the home of smoke and particulates that harm health.

Fantech and Panasonic make powerful and very quiet fans. Fantech products are extra quiet in that they are designed with a remote motor unit installed away from the actual air intake. When the motor units are installed above attic insulation the fans become barely audible in the living spaces they ventilate.

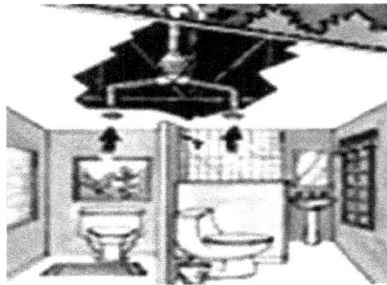

A schematic of how Fantech Fans work. Notice the motor unit sits in the attic, which makes for quiet in the house

Choose Healthy and Safe Building Materials

Design with finish materials in mind. Many building products have proven to be toxic. A solid example of toxic home environments were the FEMA (Federal Emergency Management Agency) trailers provided to Hurricane Katrina victims that proved to be so filled with formaldehyde that residents were quickly ill.

Formaldehyde is a chemical compound used in pressed woods, hard plastic/melamine dishes, and cigarette smoke. Severe and prolonged exposure can increase risk of brain cancer and leukemia. Less extreme ailments include headaches, nausea, and irritation to eyes, throat, and other soft membranes.

Avoid particle boards, plywood, and cabinets with high formaldehyde contents. Most construction requires some plywood, so make sure you use exterior grade outside only. If you must use plywood or like woods indoors make sure they are interior grade products.

PVC (poly vinyl chloride) or flexible vinyl products such as flooring, shower curtains, pipes, and some personal care products leach phthalates when heated or worn. Phthalates have been linked to breast cancer and early puberty in girls.

Never chlorinate a well. Wells are tightly plumbed and in most situations there is no way for harmful bacteria to contaminate the water. If you have a municipal water system, filter the water. Chlorine is toxic, even if low concentrations. Chlorine is linked to bladder, colon, and rectal cancers. It is also linked to increased risks of heart disease, miscarriages, and allergic reactions. If you have a septic system, or even if you don't, limit cleaning products that contain chlorine such as abrasive cleansers and dishwasher detergents. Chlorine kills or reduces the number of bacterial colonies in septic tanks that help to break down solids and keep your septic system healthy.

There are many water filtration systems on the market. Choose one that is right for your home's needs. We have a well that is heavy with iron and calcium. Toilets would turn orange, plumbing fixtures would get calcium build-up, and hair would turn a little orangey if we didn't filter out the "hard" minerals.

In short, fear the chemical world and embrace safe, organic materials. Your home will not only feel better, but so will you and your family.

Keep the following in mind: Are most of the construction and finish products environmentally sound and energy efficient? Are products recycled? Do products off-gas chemicals? Why do I need to wear gloves or a mask to install it? Are these products durable or reusable? Does installation require toxic glues or other compounds? Is this local or regional product?

Not all of us can make our homes 100% green due to material availability, lifestyle needs or choices, and costs. Green materials are often more expensive, so many of us compromise a little here and there. Consider that any green or environmentally safe construction material you choose is one less toxic material going into the home. Every little bit helps.

Style

Artfulness and architectural style should be part of your vision. Do not envision a southwestern interior with a Victorian exterior, nor an ultra modern art-deco revival exterior with Arts and Crafts interior. Your vision of the exterior and ideas for interior finished design should harmonize. Think about symmetry, asymmetry, compatible shapes, and complimentary materials. Make your house harmonize within itself and its surroundings.

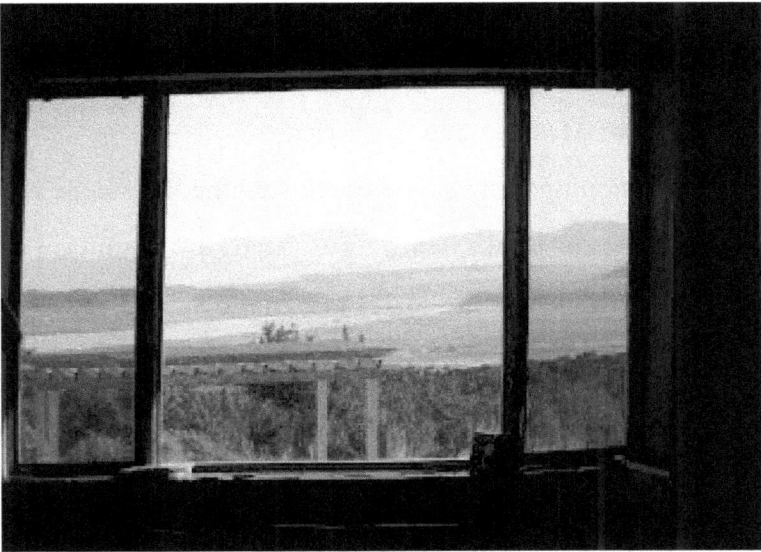

Would anyone guess that this is actually a mirror on an opposing wall reflecting the view outside?

Many straw bale homes have a southwestern theme or style to them. Mediterranean, Spanish Revival, Contemporary, Art Deco, and Ranch are just a few styles that lend themselves well to passive solar design, but any home can be heated and cooled passively.

Ask yourself if the roof's slope and design fits with the overall style of the house. While our house is essentially a southwestern ranch style, the hip roof has such a low sweeping slope, a 4:12 pitch, that it offers just a hint of an Asian pagoda. We like this, since the outside is very plain, it lends a bit of mystery as to what the interior of the house may be like. It could be decorated in minimalist Asian themes, western ranch, southwestern, or Mexican country styles.

If envisioning designs proves challenging, buy some home design magazines or books. Since I was interested in southwestern style, especially Mexican interiors, I purchased a couple nice volumes on Mexican tile and Mexican-Mission influenced architecture. Don't follow anything verbatim, but certainly mix and match features that work well together.

If you like the size of a friend's kitchen, measure it and incorporate that space into your design. If you want large walk-in showers, don't settle for what the local building center sells premade. This is your home designed by you and probably built by you to last generations, make it how and what you want it to be.

We've all seen or been in homes that are architectural works of art, but do not fit with their surroundings, or have chaotic interior floor plans. Combine functionality with artful design. Make sure designs afford a highly efficient and ultra comfortable home. Use sound and proven passive solar elements and spaces intended for human movement and pleasure, you're home will feel great.

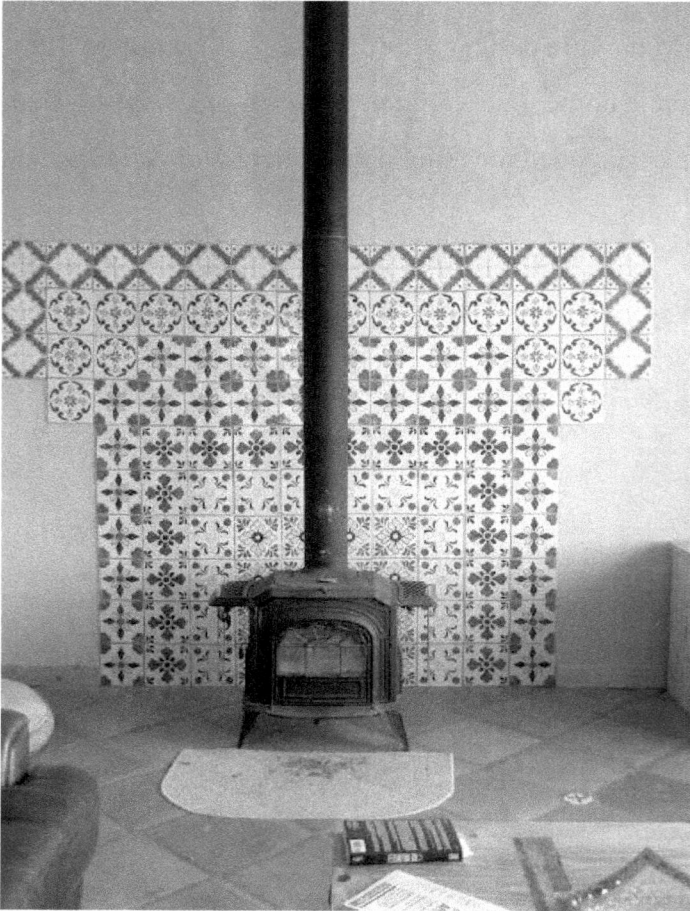

Mexican Talavera tile compliments the wood stove, protects the wall from heat, and radiates absorbed heat back into the room.

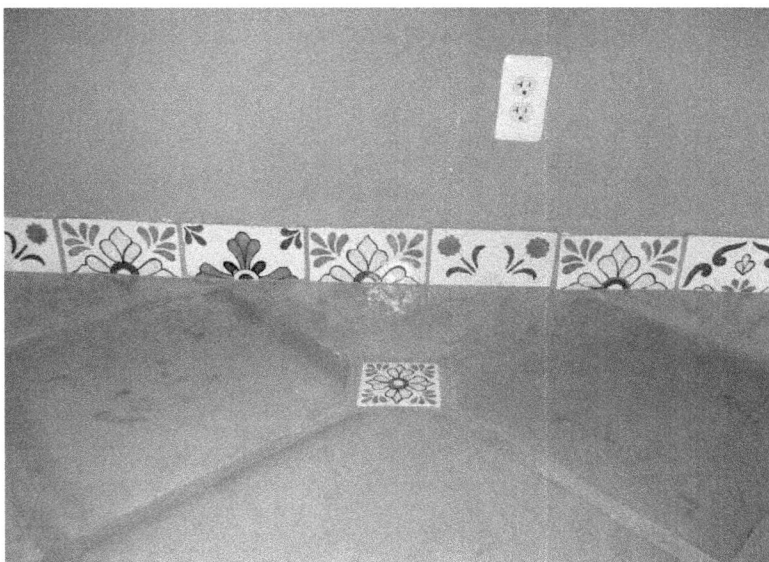

Left over tile from the wood stove back drop made for pretty base boards
in the library. Smaller accent tiles of the same pattern
were spaced throughout the Saltillo floors.

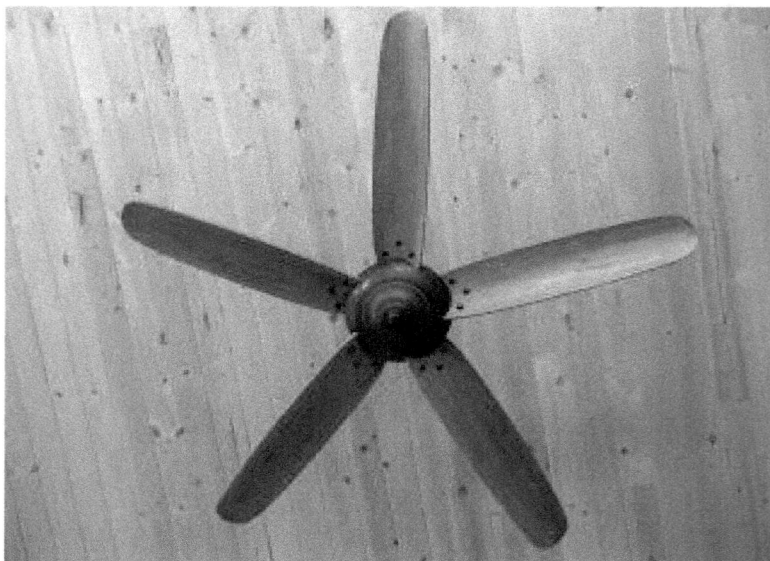

An artful and functional ceiling fan creates in warm walnut, creates a beautiful juxtaposition against the pine ceiling.

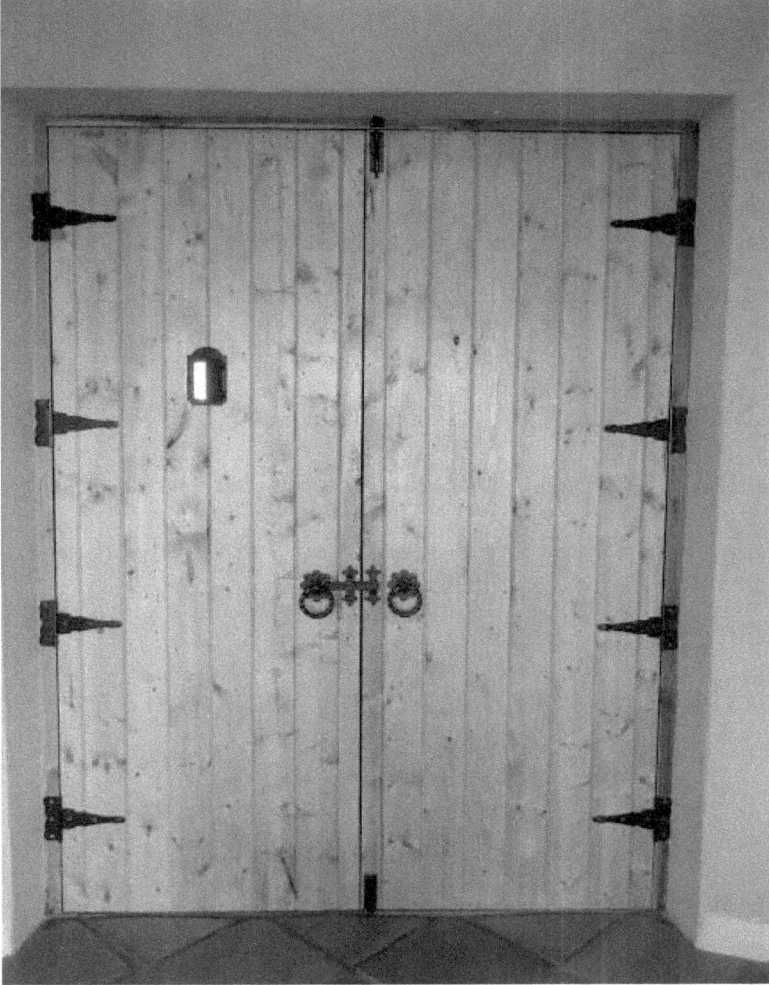

Our custom built front doors – ala Rob! The doors are tongue and groove pine on both sides and filled with rigid insulation.

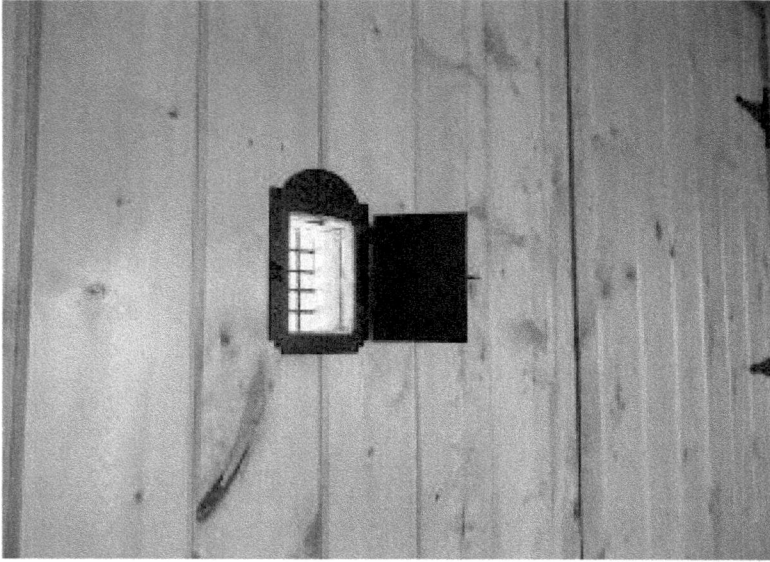

A speak-easy style peep in the front door adds personality and a bit of whimsy

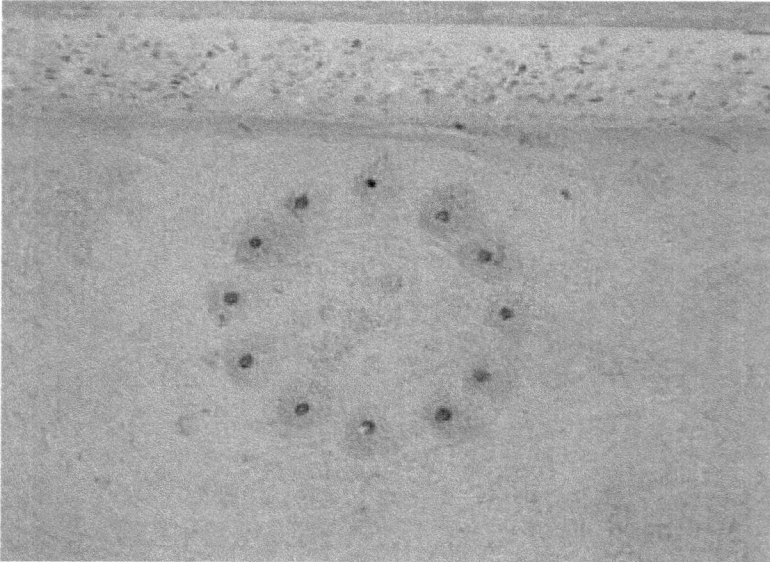

Marbles embedded in front entry steps add a little color and artfulness

Lighting

How well a house is lit affects moods and ability to perform tasks. When designing indoor lighting for energy efficiency, consider some basic design principles and methods.

For super usable lighting in rooms layer your lights. The three layers include ambient, task, and accent. This means having an overall room light or ambient light source such as recessed ceiling or other type of whole area lighting; task lighting such as a lamp or more focused recessed fixture; and lighting to create warmth or hominess in a room. Accent lighting is often achieved by well placed lamps or wall sconces.

More light or light fixtures are not necessarily better. Houses that are over lighted feel commercial, less friendly, and use power unnecessarily.

How well you see under specific lights depends on the amount of light or watts as well as the spectrum the bulb(s) put out. Cooler spectrum lighting is more suited to workshops or garages, while warmer spectrum lighting works well in homes. Cool spectrum lighting that will cast a more industrial lighting affect is typically around 4,000 degrees Kelvin. Bright white lighting is often around 3,500 degrees Kelvin, and warmer lighting less than 3000 degrees Kelvin.

Compact fluorescent lights (CFL) come in all spectrums, so you should be able to achieve high degrees of energy efficiency without using incandescent bulbs. The average lifespan of a CFL is often 6,000-15,000 hours and uses far fewer kilowatts to emit the same amount of light as an incandescent bulb. Incandescent bulbs typically last 750-1,000 hours and cost more each time you turn them on by using more kilowatts.

There's been some controversy about CFLs and mercury. When a CFL breaks in a home, landfill, or elsewhere, miniscule amounts of mercury are released - about four milligrams per bulb on average. When bulbs are intact and in use they pose no health hazards, however, they must be disposed of properly. The Environmental Protection Agency provides information on proper disposal as does the packaging in which CFLs come.

LED, or light emitting diodes, are much longer lasting than any other bulbs – up to ten times as long as CFLs. LEDs do not have filaments and are solid, they prove extremely durable. These bulbs don't emit as much heat, have no mercury, and only use 2-17 watts of electricity. LED lights are initially more expensive than CFLs, but cost is recouped over time and they produce a much more global, spherical array of light than other bulbs, so rooms or areas receive more even lighting.

Bulbs are one feature of lighting, fixtures are another. Don't plan on installing energy efficient LEDs or CFLs in "contractor's pack" recessed cans. Choose the recessed can or other fixture carefully. There are quality differences. I spent a considerable amount of time comparing recessed can lighting and ended up paying a little more for cans that are extremely low voltage draws. They were made better than the bulk priced cans and installed easily.

Again, think function or task first then style of lighting second. The work space over kitchen counters needs good task lighting, so install energy efficient recessed cans or other overhead task lights appropriately. When entertaining and creating a mood, dimmed wall sconces may work well throughout the house.

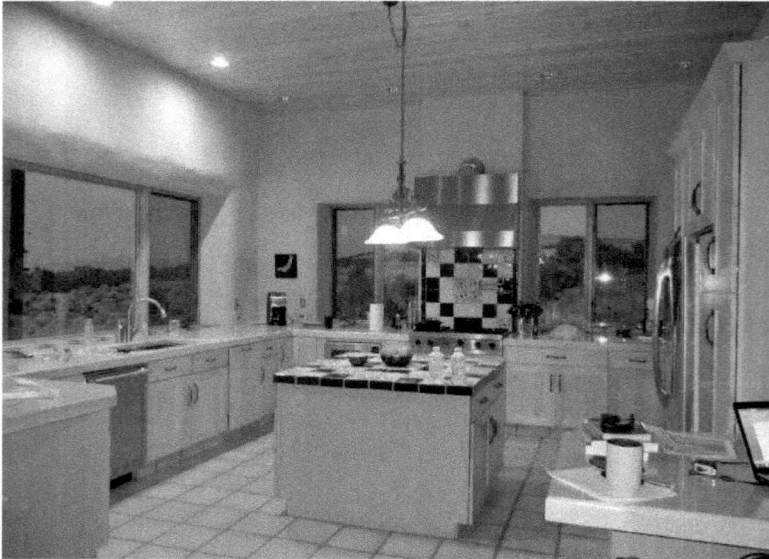

Task lighting over work surfaces is supplied with energy efficient recessed cans coupled with compact fluorescent bulbs

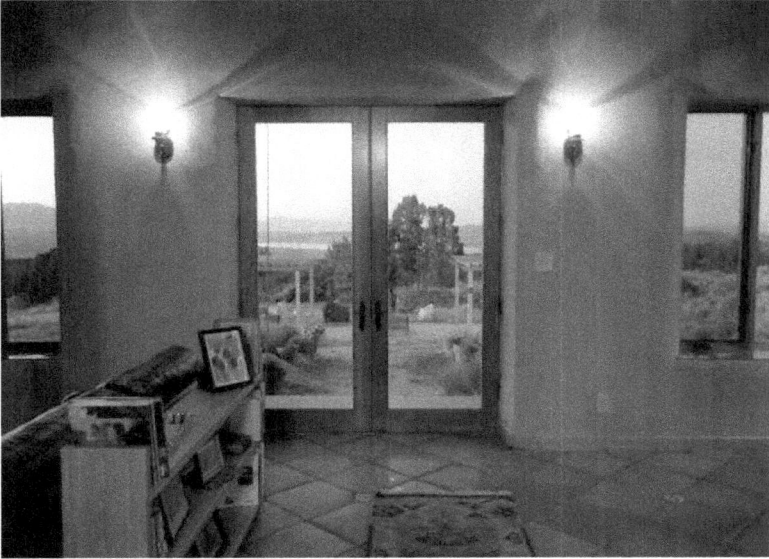

When over head energy efficient lighting is turned off, sconces on dimmer switches create a nice warm glow

Many years ago a friend of mine remodeled a very old small house. The newly installed lighting was fabulous. When I asked how he established such functional and beautiful lighting effects his response was, "Thirteen dimmer switches." There are CFL and LED fixtures that can be dimmed.

Of course the best way to save energy on lighting is to not use it. Use as much natural daylight as possible. Dark colored walls and rooms with fewer than two windows on different walls are darker and require artificial lighting more frequently. Plan smartly.

Design Check-list

_____Home's east-west axis should face as near to true south as possible

_____South facing long wall

_____7-12% of homes total sq. ft. is glazing/glass on south wall

_____Roof overhang/eave depth is appropriate for latitude

_____Breeze pathways

_____Vents exhaust to the outside

_____Thermal mass flooring considerations

_____Building is up from grade and walls adequately covered by roof design

_____Form follows function for all spaces

_____Symmetry and balance of structural and visual features

_____Windows on two sides of every room

_____No hallways

_____Storage space

_____Mechanical room

_____Kitchen and bathroom spaces are utilitarian

_____Master bedroom privacy

_____Common area, including kitchen, at the heart of the home

_____Pathways do not interrupt conversation or work areas

_____Entries are sheltered from weather

_____Entries, especially the main entry, is a separation point between outside and inside worlds

_____Ceiling heights suit their corresponding floor spaces

_____Corners and irregular angles are minimal in number

_____Materials are conserved

_____Design is appropriate for owner-builder's skill level of construction

_____Materials are sustainable and environmentally responsible

_____Finish materials are non toxic: zero volatile organic compound (VOC) paints and finishes

_____Formaldehyde free woods

_____Water conserving fixtures

_____Energy conscious room, task, and ambient lighting

Chapter 5

Drafting Home Plans

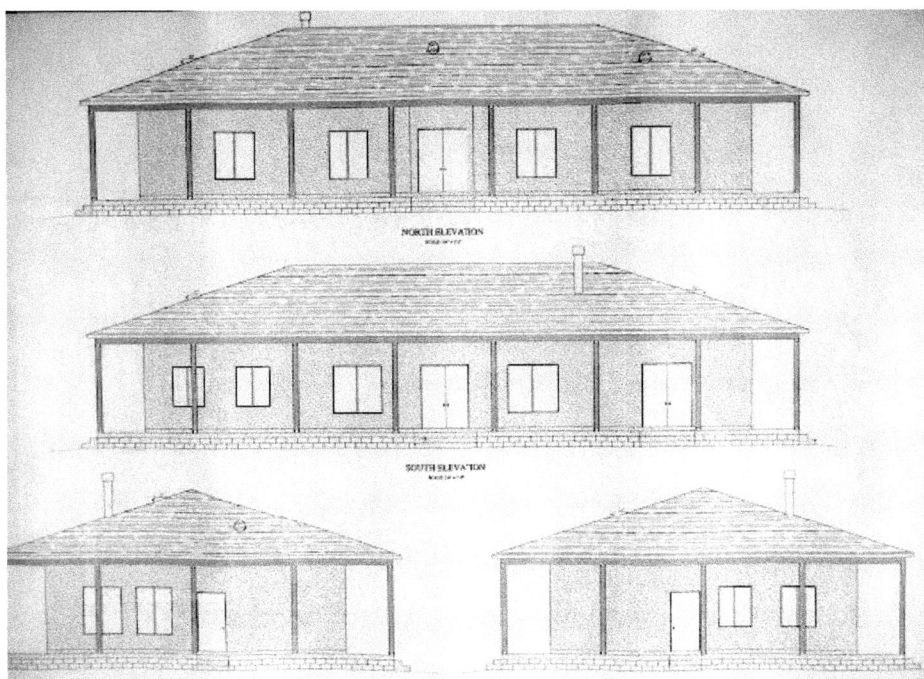

Exterior elevation drawings

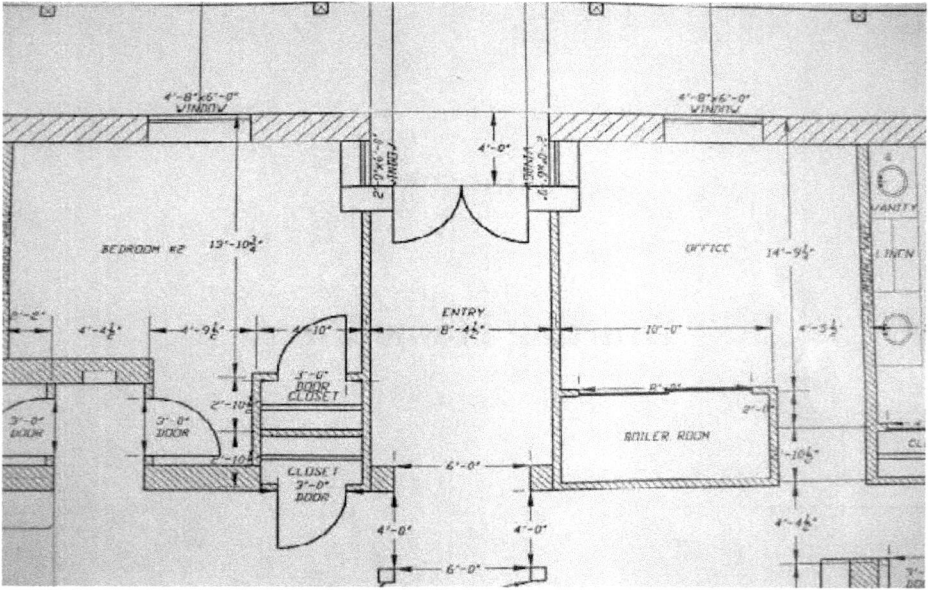

Snapshot of floor plan

I've discussed site selection, passive solar elements, green building considerations, and general principles of what makes a home comfortable and pleasing. Hopefully, you have a style in mind, so now the next step is sketching concepts to scale using graph paper. Take time. Enjoy.

Drafting a home design is a time consuming process. Meticulous and detailed planning makes for easier construction process and provides greater satisfaction with the finished home. Painstaking planning will also save money in that you'll have workable, reasonable dimensions, and be able to recycle materials whenever possible since you will have planned wisely.

Depending upon design complexity and finish materials, it's doable to build a nice house for less than current construction market prices. If using imported Italian marble, rare woods, exotic flooring, a slate roof, lots of angles and corners, or other high end options a home will cost more.

Straw bale homes are not cheaper per square foot to construct than other homes. The savings results from careful materials selection and by doing much of the construction work yourself.

I've already mentioned that the more angles or corners a home has the more labor it takes to construct, and often at greater expense and often waste. A simple rectangle or square with four corners is easier and cheaper to construct than a home with multiple wings, octagonal or dodecagonal rooms, and curved roofs. If you have unlimited funds and hiring a professional crew then the sky may be the limit on design. However, owner-builders or other do-it-yourselfers sleep better with keeping things simple and working hard.

A general rule of thumb is that for each additional corner you add, beyond the basic four add an additional 3% to the total building cost for time and materials. Corners take time to cut, form and support. Corners also take more mathematics and general carpentry skills. You know your budget and how skilled a builder you are, or have the will to become, so keep this in mind when designing.

Before sketching measure existing spaces. If you like the size of a friend's kitchen, measure it and note the dimensions. If a current shower is too small look at shower units at the local building store, or simply design a large walk-in shower that can be tiled or otherwise finish nicely. Decide how small a guest bedroom, or how large a master suite should be. Get some real world numbers to help you envision a realistic and affordable floor plan.

Next, estimate how much per square foot typical homes in your area cost to build. Knowing average cost per square foot in the areas will help you to create a design that is within your budget.

In 2006, when we began construction on our home, newer homes on an acre or two were selling for around $150 per square foot. Our materials cost for our home was just over $80 per square foot.

Begin drafting or sketching with a rough idea of the total size and shape of a home you want to build. Buy some home magazine or floor plan books to get ideas. Consider the following: 1 or 2 story? Style? Tudor? Cottage? Spanish Revival? Craftsman? Ranch? Basement? Daylight or walkout? Open airy rooms or quaint and cozy? Number of bedrooms? Library? Art room? Hobby room? Media gathering spot? Dog wash station? Bar or game room?

Drafting floor plans and elevation drawings to scale will not be done in a day, a week or likely even a few months. I worked on ours for more than two years to come up with a final design. And in actuality had home design ideas stored in my head and in file folders for years. Even after my final sketches were turned in to blue prints I made two minor changes.

Sketching takes a little practice, but with scale ruler and plenty of graph paper you'll have it down in no time. Knowing common blue print notations and creating final drafts using these notations will have drawings ready for the structural engineer. A structural engineer will create larger scaled plans with engineering specifics for you to submit to the building inspector and that you will actually use on the construction site.

Drafting Floor Plans

To begin drafting you will need some basic tools.

1. A **scale ruler** for making drawings that reflect the exact size and proportion of your structure. These are usually triangular shaped "rulers" with three sides, with two scales on each side. You will most often use the ¼" scale. ¼" on paper will represent 1" of real world measurement.

2. A ream of **graph paper** – ¼" scale works well. You can print this off of the internet at: **www.freegraphpaper.com**

3. **Pencils and sharpener**

4. A calculator. If you know you'll see this project through, then spend the money on a **construction calculator** that can convert decimals to fractions, inches and feet, feet to inches, meters to feet, calculates rise and run of slopes (roof), calculates cubic yards for concrete or other materials use and so on. A construction calculator is a great little tool.

5. **Tape measures** of varying lengths and types. I recommend a 35' Fat Max by Stanley because it holds well at extended lengths; in addition to 100' or longer reel tape measure for actually laying out a home's footprint (the area of ground it will cover); and a shorter, tape measure to keep on hand for quick smaller measurement such as counter depths and such.

6. **A protractor** may be handy for making perfectly square corners or other angles

7. **Computer Assisted design (CAD program)** if you are software savvy.

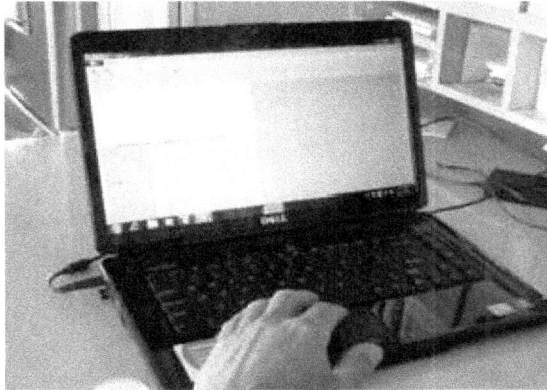

If you are well versed with Paint or other graphing and drawing programs on computer you could do all of your drafting with software.

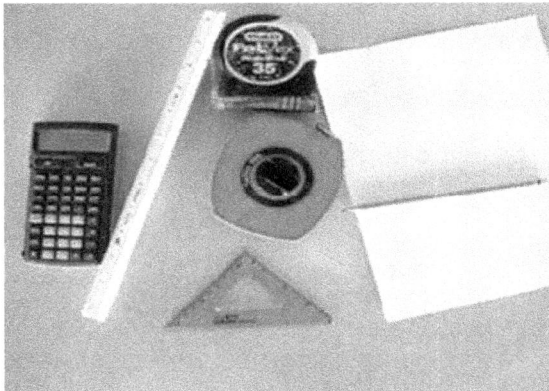

Some common drafting tools, from left: calculator, scale ruler; tape measures, protractor, graph paper, and pencil

When drawing floor plans:

• North is always the top of the page, south the bottom, east to the right, and west to the left

• Imagine you have lifted the roof off of your house and are peering in from a bird's eye view.

• All interior and exterior doors are denoted by having them opened, with their hinged side attached to the corresponding wall.

• Exterior doors open in.

• Straw bale walls have diagonal lines

• Scale carefully the differences between 2"x4" or 2"x6" walls

• Windows are marked by double lines on the exterior side, and by not being filled in with diagonal lines or other marks

• Sliding closet doors are shown closed with the meeting ends slightly overlapping and parallel to one another

• Bathroom vanity basins are ovals

• Kitchen sinks are always drawn with double basins, even if installing a single basin sink

• Bathroom fixtures are drawn as simple aerial perspectives - Standard bathroom vanity height is 34 ½"

• Standard kitchen counter height is 36h

• Standard kitchen counter depth is 24". If you have counter height windows in your kitchen your counters will appear to have greater depth due to the thickness of your straw bale walls

- Kitchen and bathroom counters are simple lines that extend from the walls they will be mounted against
- Notice that all rooms tell what they are. There are no abbreviations for specific room names in this example
- The exterior porch, outside of the straw bale walls, is marked by a simple line and post supports spaced evenly around the structure
- Standard ceiling height is 8'
- Standard door heights and widths are 80" or 6'8" and 32" or 2'8", respectively
- Windows come in many stock or standard heights and widths.
- Window shop for kitchen appliances and bathroom fixtures to obtain roughed-in dimensions. When drafting to scale you must be accurate. If you decide upon slightly different appliances or fixtures later, dimensions can be altered slightly, but plan as accurately as possible.
- For multi-story homes, or homes with basements, use a separate sheet of graph paper for each level. Make sure all structural features such as stairs and walls align to scale amongst all pages.
- Avoid plumbing straw bale walls if/when possible.

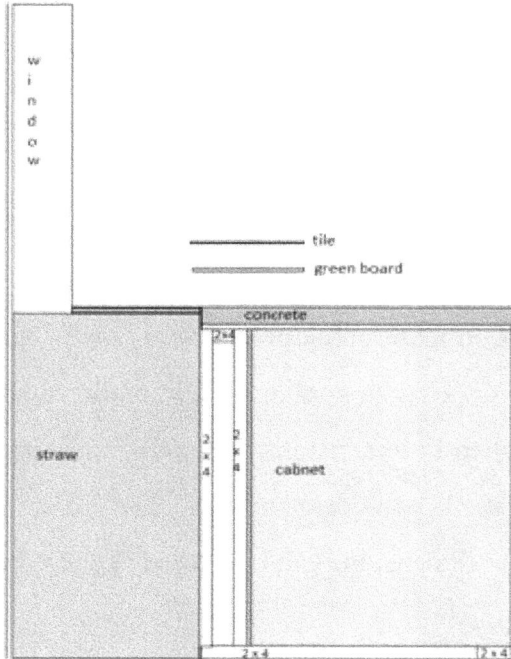

We avoided running plumbing in the straw bale wall behind the kitchen sink, and accommodated 34"d counter tops by constructing a 10" wide chase or s pace in between the baled wall and the cabinets. This space was accounted for on my initial draft

Bathtubs are commonly 60" long and 32' wide. Toilets require 30" widths as codes don't allow them too close to vanities or walls; and they require 36" of space in front of them. If a door is directly in front of a toilet, make sure the threshold is 36" away from the front of the commode.

Consider where electrical outlets will go; the National Electric Code dictates spacing and number.

Consider where main power will enter the structure for breaker box placement.

Decide where main water lines might enter the home and how the plumbing will run throughout the building. Since outdoor plumbing from a pump house or municipal source will be underground, plan accordingly with 2" conduit to protect pipes from sharp rocks or other damaging elements. The water main line may run up through concrete floor into and through a framed wall, and then into the ceiling to be directed to its destinations.

Plan to use a PEX tubing, Rehau brand is excellent quality, rather than copper, as it is very easy to work with and you can purchase blue pipes for cold water and red pipes for hot which makes running connections all the more easy. Cheap plastic pipes are just that, don't use them as they will be more prone to kinks, cracks, and freeze breaks.

Plan a utility room or boiler room for solar workings, heat exchanger tanks, flash hot water heaters, or other mechanics. It's often good to have this room fairly centrally located within the house and/or near an exterior wall. Our boiler room is completely surrounded with interior walls, so we plumbed a floor drain that runs under the slab and out to the garden– just in case we would ever have to drain the heat exchanger tank (solar hot water storage). The local building inspector will likely require such a drain through the floor or outside wall.

Incorporate a laundry room and/or mud room for washing; and perhaps a big farm sink for pet bathing.

Decide where city sewer, or septic drain lines, will exit the structure and plan accordingly.

Preliminary Drafts 1 sq. = 2ft

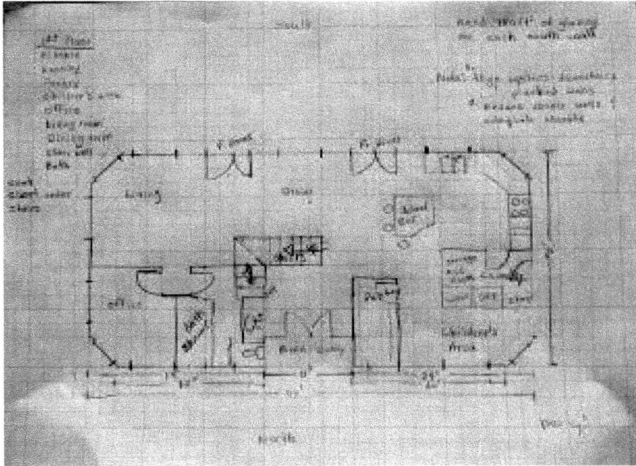

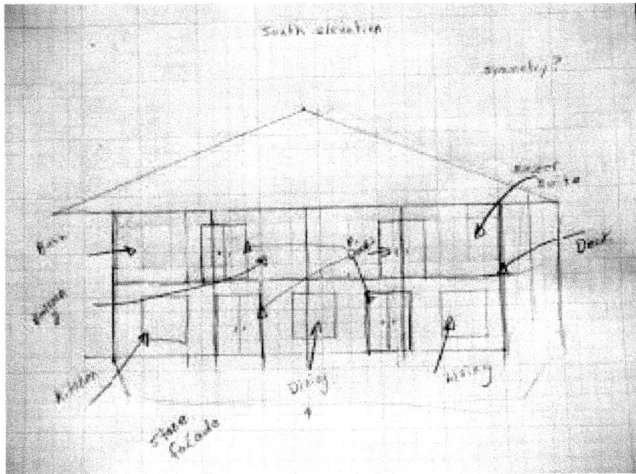

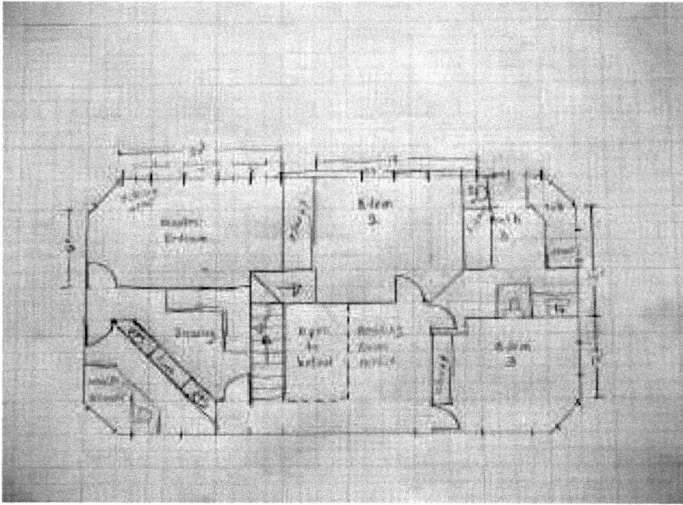

A single story home rough draft for a single or couple.

20' x 30' home 600 sq. ft.

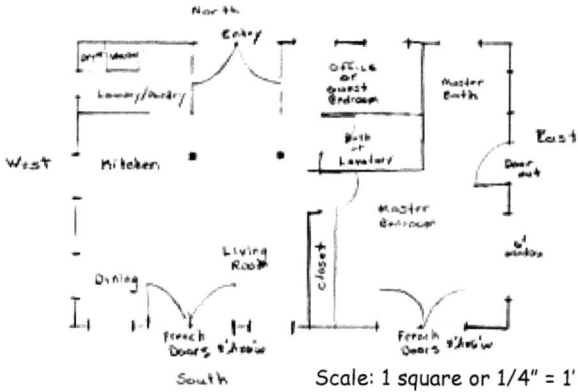

Scale: 1 square or 1/4" = 1'

Once the floor plans and exterior elevation drawings are exactly how you want them, make some copies that will allow you to code in electrical and plumbing schematics. Often engineers will provide you with blank or non-detailed floor plan drafts for this purpose.

On this note, there are some blue print elements that a lay person, owner-builder should not be responsible for within design.

They include:

Truss schematics – where rafters will fall and who they web together - these will be engineered by your local lumber yard or a structural engineer

Foundation details – how much steel, grade of concrete and footing placements – best left to structural engineer

Wiring – if you feel competent to understand local codes you may have no problem noting gauge and type of wiring.

I read code books, looked up blue print symbols and have done my own electric and plumbing schematics. Anything I was unsure about, I phoned the local county inspector's office for clarification and had no problem drafting, passive blue print inspections, and installing since we did not hire an electrician.

Plumbing – What is true for electric also goes for plumbing. If you feel competent, read the codes for your area and denote size and type of pipes.

Very few county or city building departments accept hand generated scale drawings done by someone who is not a licensed professional engineer or architect as there are structural safety issues involved with any building.

Since you'll be taking in specific, highly detailed drawings of your residence to an engineer the cost for rendering blueprints shouldn't be too much as compared to having the engineer or architect generate raw designs based upon a list of wants and descriptions.

The structural engineer will create foundation schematics to fit the floor plan with the necessary footing depths specific to local codes and soil conditions. He or she will note concrete mix requirements (3000 lb or 4000 lb are common terms), and markings for rebar placement. They will detail floor joists for crawl space foundations and all other structural and safety concerns such as size and type of seismic anchors, rebar, and so forth so that you meet code requirements and have a structure that will be safe and sound.

Concrete and steel is an amazingly strong combination. An engineered foundation plan will set your mind at ease if you live in earthquake prone areas. Analysts 2010 earthquake that devastated Haiti reported that if the concrete homes had had steel reinforcement, i.e. rebar, there wouldn't have been as many collapsed structures and many fewer deaths.

A sound structure will afford you a good night's sleep.

The engineer will also develop a roof truss schematic. You will not design and build roof rafters or ceiling joists yourself as most building inspectors require an engineer's stamp on these as well.

Trusses will be built by a lumber company and brought on a large truck that will slide them off onto the ground. You will have to lift them on to the top of your walls or beams on your own, unless they have excessively long spans, where you may have to hire a crane operator to lift them.

Some lumber yards or lumber companies offer a truss drafting service when they bid on the lumber for your home. Once the engineering team had completed our blue prints, the lumber yard's truss engineers altered the truss schematic slightly. This was fine, as we paid nothing additional for this service.

If any professional you interview tells you they have no experience with straw bale, rammed earth, or other natural yet structurally proven natural homes , or are unwilling to work with you based upon an initial phone conversation, request a meeting to show your designs. This may eliminate the fear of the unknown factor that your local professional may feel.

Engineers or architects should charge you a flat rate. Avoid any professional who wants to charge by the square foot. Typically their first piece of advice is to make the home larger.

Drafting Exterior Elevations

Exterior elevation drawings will be to scale and accurately reflect windows, doors, chimneys, skylights, and other interior/exterior features. Your elevation drawings will include:

• All four sides of the exterior of your home

• Basement depth below grade

• How your roof will look

• Generally reflect the exterior appearance and material choices

Below and following page: all four elevations, west, east, north, and south home, as well as the garage elevations which are on one page. In the south elevation sketch, all windows, with the exception of French doors, were later made wider. Completely accurate representations of finish materials in elevations drawings are not necessary as the larger purposes of elevation drawings are to establish heights, widths, overall appearances, and elevation from grade.

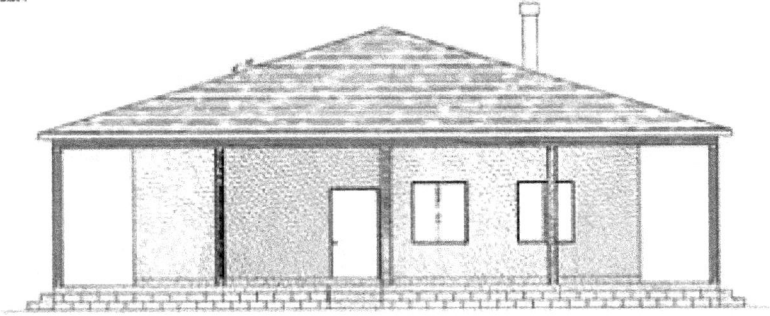

WEST ELEVATION

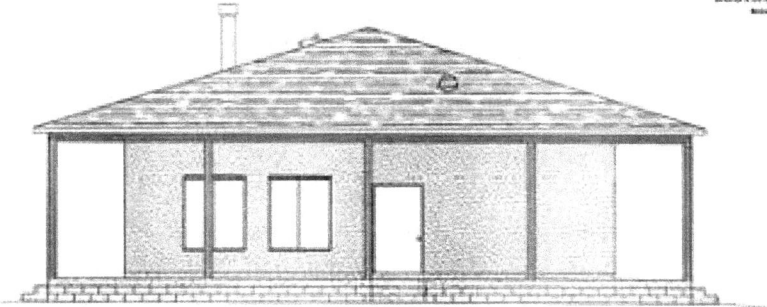

EAST ELEVATION

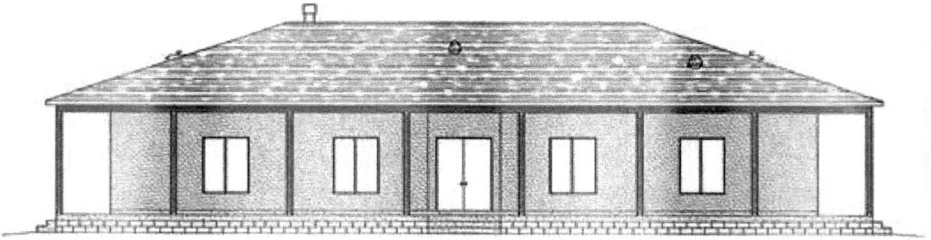

NORTH ELEVATION
SCALE 1/4" = 1'-0"

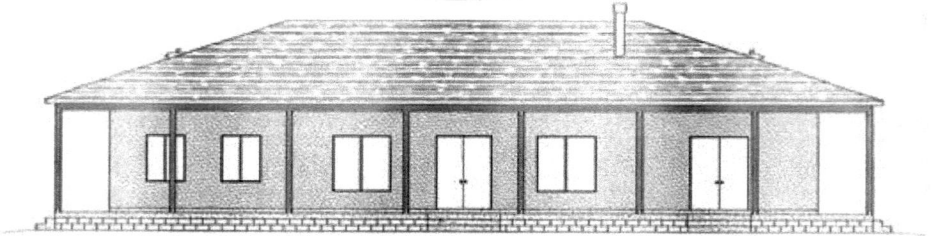

SOUTH ELEVATION
SCALE 1/4" = 1'-0"

Notice that in all these elevation sketches, the home is 2' above grade. Concrete masonry units (blocks) that are actually the upper part of the foundation stem wall are exposed, yet still penetrate in excess of 3' below grade.

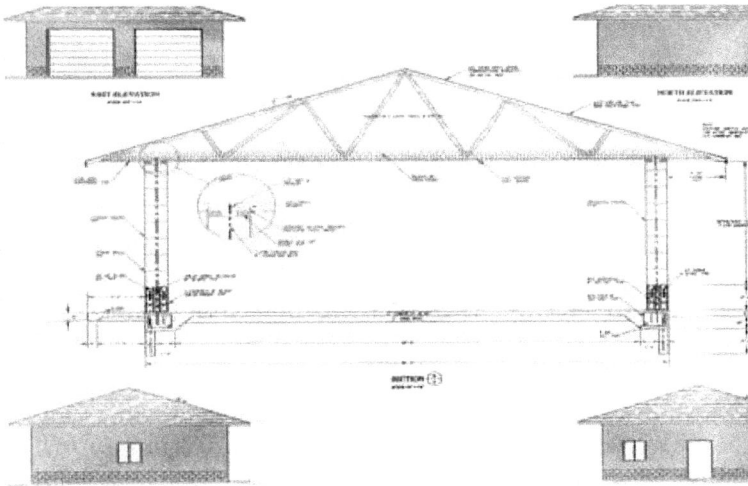

Garage structure different from house in that there is no elevated porch.

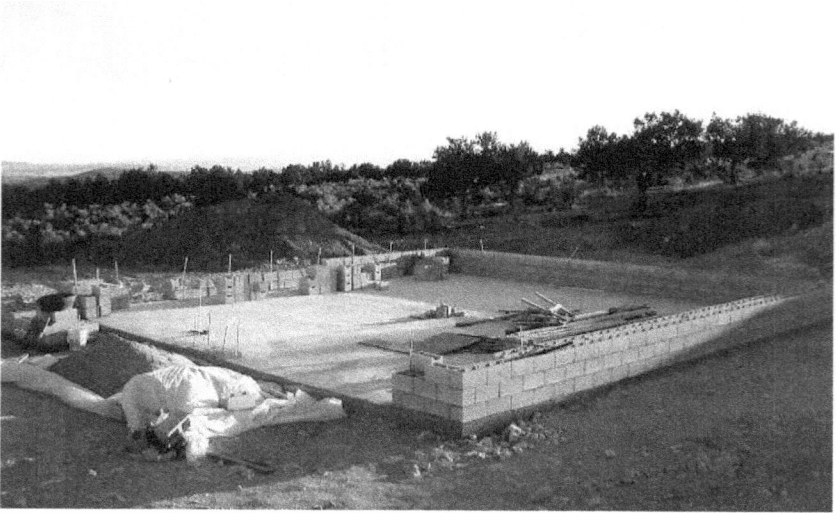

Garage foundation slab and 24"h 18"w base wall

Remember the two major considerations with straw bale homes are to keep them *up and covered*. So if you choose to build on a slab make sure you either live in a dry climate where rain and snow are light, or that you raise the height of your finished floor well above finished grade so that when rain or snow does come they do not saturate lower portions of exterior walls.

Drive around neighborhoods and look at roof lines and slopes. How steep does a roof in your area need to be? Are there heavy snow loads or no snow at all? What fits well with the style of your house? How steep a slope feels safe and comfortable to work on?

Don't let anyone tell you that you can't alter plans once the building inspector has approved them. You can, but try not to. It will cost more money at the county office.

We didn't have to get approval from the inspector's office to alter the position of non-load bearing walls or doorways, but we did need to submit information when we changed the size of a kitchen window and needed a beefier header above it. Our engineers submitted the paper work and it cost us $40 at the county office.

Be as articulate as possible and firm in design justifications with the engineers. They will likely be used to drafting stock tract type homes that are not necessarily ergonomically designed or as well thought out as the drafts you offer. When they question design details explain your rationale and thinking for them. More often than not, they'll jump in and help you to improve what's already pretty good.

With rural building sites, a county office may require that a septic permit first before they review plans and issue a building permit. You also may be required to have two building permits, one for the house and one for the garage, if they are separate structures.

With building permit and good blue prints in hand you will be ready to stake out your footprint and begin construction – maybe. If you need to secure a construction loan for your project now is the time to do it.

Chapter 6

Financing and Permits

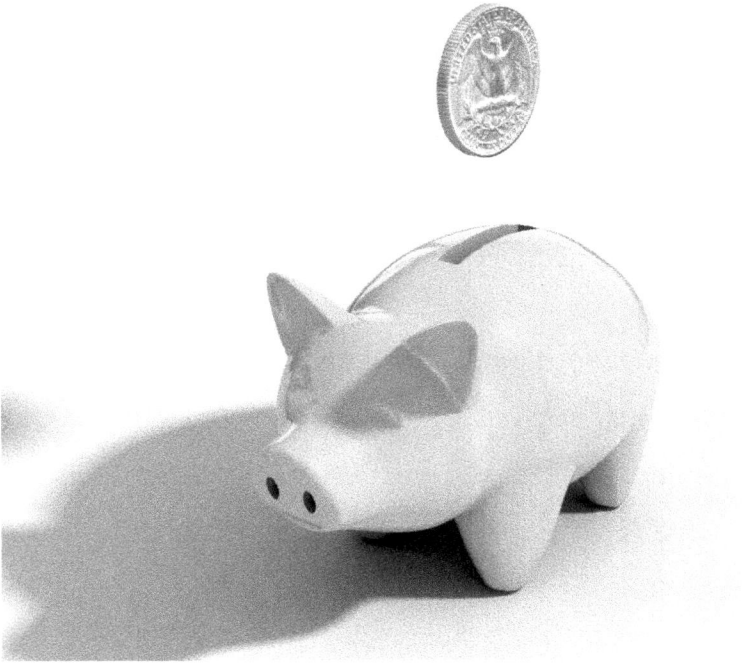

The best way to finance construction is with cash – yours. If you can pay cash you will be debt free, have no construction dead line, and probably experience fewer headaches during the construction process.

Owner-builder construction loans can be difficult to obtain, especially after the recent mortgage crisis. Though as of this update, 2013, construction money is becoming available again as the housing market is recovering.

You may be asked to document all construction experience that you have had in order to prove that you have something of what it takes to complete an entire home project. If an owner-builder has never done any construction, it may be difficult to get a construction loan. Don't cave-in if a lender insists upon you hiring a contractor. A contractor will take 20% or more of the construction budget. Shop around for another lender that offers true owner-builder loans. Private money may also be an option, finding a private individual in your area who lends to contractors or owner-builders. These people often charge higher interest though, so be careful. The best bet, if you've never built anything before and have the time, is to start getting some construction experience. Work part time for a contractor or developer. Gain some experience, then seek the loans.

Another alternative is to concede to some hired labor. Maybe you can find a contractor who will agree to help with foundation, oversee your project, and sign off on the bank papers. In one case I know, the contractor dictated exactly how to do every step, according to the owner-builder's plans, and simply would come by to see if things were done right. The owner builder could also phone the contractor with questions. That situation worked out well.

Look on the internet. Ask other people you know who have built or may be building. It may take months to find financing, but you will find it.

The bank or financial institution financing the project will ask for similar documentation as if applying for a mortgage. The process takes time and you'll have to jump through hoops, often producing the same documentation of income(s) or banking histories more than once. Don't get discouraged for frustrated.

Banks will want to see that you have some savings and that your land is free and clear of debt, liens, or loans. In the old days, banks might have wrapped land payments into construction loan, but in today's market this would be an extremely rare exception. Having land free and clear is similar to applying for a mortgage and having a nice down payment. Lenders want some equity so they are not loaning 100% of the total value of the project.

A lender will require copies of materials' bids. Submit copies of blue prints to local lumber suppliers, home building centers, electrical supply stores, plumbing supply companies, and/or roofing contractors to get lists of the cost of each material needed. This means that you will have to have a close idea of all the rough and finish materials you will want to use in the house so your bids will be accurate. Don't obtain a bid for cheap Formica counter tops if you plan to install granite, or you'll end up short of funds in your construction loan.

Getting bids on materials is also wise practice if you are paying out of pocket. You'll want to know where the best deals can be had.

Scrutinize each bid. We took our blue prints to our local big box home improvement center which said they'd have the completed bid back to us within two weeks. A month later they apparently had lost our blue prints. After a handful of telephone calls from me to store managers they found the prints and the bid – which cost me $160. I stood at the "Building Professionals" desk in the store and leafed through the bid quickly, then finally told them that the materials list was completely wrong. They had mixed up somewhere and given me someone else's construction supply list, yet it had my name attached. The store refunded my $160. Needless to say, we purchased most of our lumber from another supplier.

The bank will higher, at your expense, an appraisal service to appraise your land and blue prints together to determine an estimate of what the home will be worth upon completion. You don't want this valuation to be too great otherwise the bank will think you can't afford to build the house you planned. You also don't want the appraisal to come back too low, or you won't get all the money you need to build, and may have to make materials or size concessions.

Most completed owner built homes appraise for more than their cost to build. Even with the housing market crisis during the time we built, our home still appraised for approximately 30% more than we had into it, not counting our labor.

Lenders stipulate time limits – usually one year. They will grant extensions if a project is not finished, but extensions cost. We paid a lot out of pocket for extensions plus the extra interest on the construction loan during the time we spent building. Construction loan interest is always higher than a typical mortgage rate.

Plan well. Work fast. Work hard every day until the house is finished. That's what it takes to finish a home in a somewhat timely manner. Most people don't want to take ten years building.

When beginning construction, establish payment accounts with the local lumber yard and other suppliers where you obtained bids. Order materials just before they're needed, and then every month or two complete a "Construction Draw Request", which is document attached to receipts requesting payment from the lender to be made directly to the materials' suppliers. Often, lenders will set limits on the number of draws during the construction process. It's nice to pay bills every month, but if you're limited to eight draws in a year's time, it means that some months suppliers may have to wait for their money. Compare the cost between the suppliers' late penalties and the lenders additional draw fee, and decide upon the lesser evil. If paying cash for materials and you need reimbursement from the lender, show all receipts duly noting that the account was paid.

Construction loans cover materials and if you budgeted for it, labor. The loans will not pay for tools. You'll buy your own tools and rent larger pieces of equipment as necessary. Watch for sales. It's difficult to give a precise estimate of what tools will cost, but avoid the mistake we made of renting a backhoe, or other heavy equipment for extended lengths of time, especially if you live rurally and suspect you'll use it more over the years to come; or you can even sell it after a project is completed. We spent enough money renting a backhoe as it would have taken to buy a good used one. This was our only financial mistake on the project. We just had no idea how much rock we would encounter when excavating or all the continued need for a backhoe after the foundation was dug.

Itemize tools for each phase of construction. Estimate a few thousand dollars for good quality tools, such as ladders, nail gun(s), a cement mixer, and a decent laser level. If land area is rocky and excavation work appears extensive it will likely be wise to buy a backhoe, or hire a backhoe operator, as renting can run in the tens of thousands of dollars.

As you progress through various construction phases the lender will likely require inspections after specific phases before they will issue more checks or authorize more payments for materials. This is often never a problem. Just phone the lender when you've completed the specific phase and they'll order an inspector to come out and verify.

This said, we did run into a rather inept inspector. He had zero experience with straw bale homes. The lender required an inspection after drywall was completed. We had some interior framed walls sheathed with drywall and some ceilings as well. I phoned the lender to tell them our drywall was completed. Actually, Rob was putting the finishing tape on the laundry room so the drywall work was 98% complete.

After the inspector came to inspect the dry wall phase he reported to the lender that the dry wall was only 10% complete. I had explained to him that the interior face of the straw bale walls would not be covered in drywall, but rather lime plastered. The lender questioned us as if we were thieving. Needless-to-say I took plenty of photos and immediately forwarded them to the lender to prove my point. They released funds within a few days. I also requested that from that point on the lender use a different, more savvy and up-to-date home inspector.

Once a home is complete, the local inspector's office will issue a Certificate of Occupancy, commonly referred to as a C.O. This will be the document needed to begin the process of converting the construction loan into a regular mortgage. The bank will likely also require an independent inspector to make sure everything is completed as some counties will issue C.O.s if the kitchen and at least one bathroom are finished. This hardly constitutes a completely finished home – especially in the eyes of a lender.

During construction, keep credit scores up and debts low, otherwise obtaining financing may be more difficult.

Building Permits

Building permits are generally issued by the county or city building inspector's office. Just phone them or stop by for what they require. Typically as long as you have engineer stamped blue prints you shouldn't have any problem obtaining the permit(s). A permit application will ask your name, parcel number, legal description, job site physical address, owner's name(s), and contractor's name. You can be the contractor or check the box for owner-builder. You will submit this application, with the appropriate fee, and two copies of the blue prints. The building inspector's office will keep one set on file and give you back a stamped approved copy to keep on hand at the job site.

If you are doing all the work yourself, you will likely sign off as the builder or contractor, electrician, and plumber. The inspector's office will also require electrical and plumbing schematics. These are separate, simplified floor plan prints with the electrical icons and plumbing symbols noted. The engineers we hired to turn our scale drawings into blue prints gave me a copy of the icons and plumbing symbols so I signed off as the electrician and plumber once I had completed the plan schematics. It was relatively easy. Electrical and plumbing code books come in handy to specify gauge of wire and type of pipes – but that's really about it. These are very straightforward for a common home.

If your home and garage are separate buildings two separate permits will likely be issued, one for each structure. The fee for permits is based upon total square footage. I believe the total fee for both our garage and house permits was around $400.

With permits in hand and financing secured, you may begin construction. Some lenders may require a copy of the building permit before they finalize a loan, but all lenders are different.

Conclusion

I hope I have clarified some of the thoughts and processes that DIY home design and building entails. Take time in planning so that no small detail gets overlooked. Careful planning and thought about how you live daily will result in the best home design. It's not rocket science and you can do it. Be resourceful. If you feel uncomfortable or insecure about a design or construction decision, consult with someone knowledgeable, do some research, or e-mail me and we'll troubleshoot.

Planning, designing, and building your own home will prove mentally and physically gratifying. Fear not, and venture forth. You will be fine and your home will be fabulous.

Acknowledgements

Special thanks to Rob for offering technical information, knowing how to build everything well, and for being a great partner in life. Love to Kevin and Mike, my sons, who on occasion would drive five hours to lend us helping hands in stuccoing, installing water lines, or other work, and putting up with Gulag-like conditions. Thanks to Jennifer McKelvey, graphic designer, and Kevin's wonderful partner, who helped with layout so that this book could happen sooner rather than later.

Bibliography

Alexander, Christopher. Et al. *A Pattern Language*. New York. Oxford University Press, 1977.

Chiras, Daniel. *The Natural House*. Vermont. Chelsea Green Publishing Company, 2000.

Corum, Nathaniel. *Building a Straw Bale House*. New York. Princeton Architectural Press, 2005.

Kachadorian, James. *The Passive Solar House*.Vermont. Chelsea Green Publishing Company, 1997.

Lacinski, Paul. Bergeron, Michel. *Serious Straw Bale*. Vermont. Chelsea Green Publishing Company, 2000.

Magwood, Chris. Mack, Peter. Therrien, Tina. *More Straw Bale Building*. Briitish Columbia, Canada. New Society Press.2005.

McMenamin, Donna. *Mexican Style Interiors*.Atlglen, Pennsylvania. Schiffer Publishing Ltd., 2002.

Steen, Athena Swentzell. Steen, Bill. Bainbridge, David. *The Straw Bale House*.Vermont. Chelsea Green Publishing Company, 1994.

Steen, Bill and Athena. *The Beauty of Straw Bale Homes*. Vermont.
Cheslea Green Publishing, 2000.

Susanka, Sarah. *The Not So Big House*. Newtown, Connecticut. The Taunton Press, 2001.

Takahashi, Masako. *Mexican Tiles*. San Francisoco, California. Chronicle Press, 2000.

Witynski, Karen. Carr, Joe. *Adobe Details*.Layton, Utah. Gibbs Smith, 2002.

Witynski, Karen. Carr, Joe. *Mexican Country Style*. Layton, Utah. Gibbs Smith, 1997.

Yudelson, Jerry. *Green Building A to Z*. British Columbia, Canada/ New Society Publishers, 2007.